# ALCOHOL
# AND THE
# PUBLIC HEALTH

A study by a working party of the Faculty of Public Health
Medicine of the Royal Colleges of Physicians on the
prevention of harm related to the use of alcohol and other
drugs

D0928624

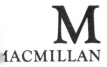

**M**
**MACMILLAN**

in association with the
Faculty of Public Health Medicine
Royal Colleges of Physicians

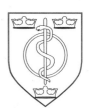

First published 1991

Published by
MACMILLAN EDUCATION LTD
Houndmills, Basingstoke, Hampshire RG21 2XS
and London
Companies and representatives
throughout the world

Edited and typeset by Povey/Edmondson
Okehampton and Rochdale, England

Printed in Great Britain by
Billing & Sons Ltd
Worcester



British Library Cataloguing in Publication Data
Faculty of Public Health Medicine
Alcohol and the public health
1. Alcoholism & drug abuse. Medical aspects
I. Title
616.86
ISBN 0–333–54778–0 (hardcover)
ISBN 0–333–54779–9 (paperback)

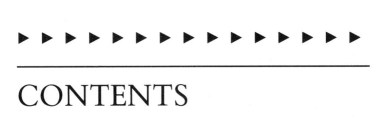

# CONTENTS

alcohol levels; Drinking pedestrian or drinking driver; The history of breath testing in the United Kingdom; Deterring the drinking driver; Breath testing; Indiscriminate systematic breath testing; Lowering the legal limit; Zero legal limit; Organisations campaigning on alcohol and road safety; Driving licence withdrawal; Host liability; Hip flask defence; Insurance schemes; Characteristics of drink drivers; Problem drinker/high risk offenders; Courses for drink-drive offenders; Prevention; Driving instruction

The need for services for problem drinkers; A range of services; Self help and family support; Alcohol and voluntary organisations; Alcoholics Anonymous; Specialist alcohol voluntary agencies; Relevant non-alcohol-specialist agencies; Alcohol problems and primary care; Alcohol and occupational health; Alcohol and general hospitals; Care of problem drinkers by psychiatric services; A planned and integrated service

Levels of prevention; Primary prevention is not enough; Local policy and strategy statements; Examples of local action; Collection of local data; Alcohol education in schools; Local work with young people; Providing alternatives; Workplace policies; Local licensing forums; Drinkwise campaigns; Local work with ethnic minorities; Local working with offenders; Prison and after-care; Alcohol and the homeless; Drying-out facilities; Meetings to elicit and co-ordinate local action

Social responsibility; Financial support for alcohol agencies; Customer education; Packaging and labelling; Health warnings on containers; Non-alcoholic drinks; Advertising; Sports sponsorship; The drinking environment

▶ ▶ ▶ ▶ ▶ ▶ ▶ ▶ ▶ ▶ ▶ ▶ ▶ ▶ ▶ ▶

# INTRODUCTION

## ▶ What is public health?

Public health medicine is concerned with maintaining and improving the health of the population by identifying and tackling the factors in our lifestyle and environment which threaten health. When the speciality was founded the greatest scourges of the population were infectious diseases whose spread was fostered by bad and unsanitary housing, polluted water supplies and food which was inadequate in quantity and quality. These dangers have now been contained (though not abolished) and the major threats to public health are posed by a different set of diseases which are fostered by another set of environmental hazards.

## ▶ Why alcohol?

There have been many previous reports on the effects of alcohol on health but these have largely concentrated on the health of individuals. Alcohol problems are very much public health problems since the health and well-being of individuals are affected not only by their own drinking but also by the drinking of their family, friends, workmates and other members of the community in which they live.

The reduction of alcohol-related problems will not be achieved entirely by the actions of individuals, though each individual has considerable influence over their own susceptibility to the hazards of the environment in which they live. Public health measures are needed to minimise the harms related to the use of alcohol in our society.

1

## ▶ Definitions

Discussion of the effects of alcohol on society are confused by the lack of agreed definitions for basic terms. In this report we use two terms:

A *heavy drinker* is defined as a man who drinks more than 50 units of alcohol per week or a woman who drinks more than 35 units of alcohol per week.

A *problem drinker* is defined as an individual whose physical, mental or social well-being has been harmed as a consequence of their drinking.

A unit of alcohol is 8 grammes, which is contained in half a pint (290 ml) of normal strength (4%) beer or lager, one single measure (1/6 gill) of spirits; or one glass (125 ml) of wine. One sixth of a gill is the standard single measure of spirits served in England. In Scotland it is one fifth of a gill and in Northern Ireland one quarter gill. (1 gill = 143 ml). Consumption of less than 21 units of alcohol per week by men or less than 14 units per week by women is generally agreed to be associated with low risk of harm.

The term 'alcoholic' is only used in this report when quoting other reports which have used it. The use of this term in the past has caused difficulties because it is so poorly defined.

## ▶ Synopsis

### Chapter 1

The consumption of alcoholic beverages has a long history in the British Isles. Consumption is now nearly double what it was fifty years ago but much less than was drunk in the eighteenth century famed for the evils of Gin Lane. Drinking is so closely interwoven with our way of life that it can be difficult to disentangle its effects, good or bad. However, alcohol consumption in the United Kingdom is less than in many continental countries and the corresponding alcohol related harm also appears to be less.

Chapter 2

Today alcohol adds considerably to the burden of ill-health on the community, making a substantial contribution to mortality and ill-health, as seen in users of hospital in-patient, casualty and general practitioner services. Alcohol is also the cause of considerable psychiatric illness.

Chapter 3

The association of drinking with criminal activity has given rise to much speculation as to whether one is caused by the other. Similarly, an association of alcohol with family disharmony and social dysfunction suggests that alcohol could also be damaging the public well being in these areas. Alcohol problems in the workplace affect both the welfare of the employee and the profitability of the business.

Alcohol problems are not restricted to the minority who drink very heavily; they also affect the much larger numbers who drink more moderate amounts. This has led to the conclusion that alcohol should be viewed as a risk factor and that a population strategy should be adopted to reduce the levels of alcohol consumed and thus the risk levels of everyone.

Chapter 4

Information is necessary for the exercise of informed choice by the individual. Clear guidelines are needed on how much people can drink without risking their health. The generally agreed guidelines of 21 units per week for men and 14 units per week for women are of course arbitrary but nevertheless serve a useful purpose. The individual also needs information on the alcohol content of drinks and the effects of alcohol on the body.

Recognising the need for individual choice does not deny society's responsibility for the health of its members. Differing emphasis on the roles of the individual and society are reflected in different models of health education and different approaches to prevention of alcohol related problems.

Whatever health education approach is adopted there is a need for evaluation. The advantages and disadvantages of different approaches such as single focus events (for example, Drinkwise

Day); sustained campaigns (for example, Tyne Tees Area Alcohol Education Campaign); coverage of alcohol issues in personal and social education in schools; alcohol coverage in multi-issues campaigns (for example, Look After Your Heart!); and media campaigns are explored. Whatever methods are adopted they need adequate funding and to date this has been notably lacking.

## Chapter 5

It is a recurrent theme of this report that while individuals are responsible for their own drinking behaviour this approach alone is unlikely to have much impact on the frequency of alcohol-related problems. It must be supported by public policy measures to reduce alcohol consumption.

One important strategy for controlling consumption of alcohol now is regulation by licensing of the times and places at which alcohol can be purchased. There is considerable debate over the efficacy of this approach but general agreement is that licensing laws are not effective if they are not enforced. Opening hours in Scotland were relaxed 10 years ago and there was no massive increase in disorder or alcohol related disease.

The recent experience of Poland and Finland and the experience in the United Kingdom after the introduction of licensing laws during the First World War suggest that decreasing the number of retail outlets decreases consumption.

Sale of alcohol to young persons under the age of eighteen is prohibited in this country, though the law is poorly enforced. Other countries have higher age limits and in countries where the age limit has been reduced the change was followed by an increase in indicators of alcohol related problems in the young.

The consumption patterns for alcohol are changing. Once, drinking was predominantly a male activity and pubs were male preserves. Now efforts are being made to make pubs more attractive to the whole family and alcohol is sold through non-specialist off-licence outlets, so making it more accessible to women. Alcohol consumption by women is increasing and these trends are likely to be accompanied by an increase in the frequency of problem drinking by women.

Local Licensing Benches have the task of administering the licensing law and issuing licences to retail alcohol. There is wide variation in the practice of different Licensing Benches and there is a need to develop consistent licensing policies which take due account of public health issues as well as public order issues.

## Chapter 6

Manipulation of the price of alcohol is one important tool for controlling alcohol consumption. There is abundant evidence that alcohol consumption is affected by the price of the product and the income of the purchaser. Wine and spirit consumption are most affected by changes in these variables, and beer to a lesser extent.

Alcohol taxes are a major source of government revenue and an increase in taxation will increase revenue since any fall in volume consumed is offset by the increased revenue per unit volume. Alcohol taxation also has the advantage that the indirect costs of consumption (the alcohol-related harms) are thereby passed to the consumer rather than to society in general. Taxation could also contribute to the public health through differential taxation on extra strength beverages. Removal of alcohol from the formula used to calculate the Retail Price Index would be helpful.

While current taxation policy on alcohol is far from satisfactory it is better than in many European countries, where alcohol is deliberately kept cheap. There is anxiety that harmonisation of taxes within the European Community could lead to a reduction in the price of alcohol in the United Kingdom with a consequent rise in consumption and increase in alcohol-related harm.

## Chapter 7

Drinking is a major cause of road traffic accidents. One third of drivers killed have blood alcohol levels above the legal limit and alcohol is implicated in a quarter of all fatal accidents. The risk of accident is increased at blood alcohol levels which are far below the legal limit of 80mg/100ml and the risk is particularly increased in young drivers.

The legal limit of blood alcohol was introduced in the Road Safety Act of 1967. The Blennerhassett Committee in 1976 reviewed the operation of the Act and proposed a series of amendments including the introduction of evidential breath testing, less emphasis on the procedural requirements for testing, and a requirement for high risk offenders to demonstrate that they have controlled the underlying problem before regaining their licence. These proposals have been implemented but other proposals relating to the powers of a police officer to require a test have not.

The chance of being detected when committing the offence of driving with blood alcohol above the legal limit remain low. There are strong arguments for introducing powers to allow both 'unfettered discretional' breath testing and 'indiscriminate systematic' breath testing (popularly known as random testing).

Other legislative changes which might reduce the problem of drink driving include reducing the legal limit and possibly more severe sentences for offenders. There are a number of organisations campaigning for the introduction of these changes. Drink-drive offenders are predominantly young, male and typically have blood alcohol levels nearly twice the legal limit. They are twice as likely as the general population to have committed other driving offences and a disturbingly high proportion have no licence. It is clear that the problem of drink drive offending is far too prevalent and that current measures have failed to resolve the problem. Public attitudes have changed and drink-driving is no longer socially acceptable, but legislation does not yet fully reflect the growing public demand for adequate protection against the danger to road safety posed by drivers who drink alcohol.

Chapter 8

Prevention is important but it does not remove the need for services to help those who are already problem drinkers. The majority of heavy drinkers will adopt safer drinking patterns without any outside intervention, and public policies must support and encourage them in this process. Others may need more intensive help and there are a range of organisations to help them. Alcoholics Anonymous is one of the oldest self-help organisations and has transformed the life of many problem drinkers although its approach may not suit everyone. Specialist alcohol agencies such as local alcohol advisory centres offer counselling for problem drinkers and support to other caring professionals. Non-specialist agencies such as Relate and the Samaritans also encounter a large number of clients with drinking problems and may offer appropriate interventions.

General practitioners, primary care teams and occupational health services have many opportunities to recognise and help patients with risky drinking patterns. General hospital staff also see many patients who have risky drinking patterns; they should recognise such patients and offer simple interventions. A very small minority of those with alcohol problems will need psychiatric treatment, possibly as an in-patient. Specialist psychiatric alcohol treatment units should be seen as under-pinning a system of helping agencies rather than as a point of first referral.

There is need for a wide range of services to meet the wide range of types and severity of alcohol-related problems. These services need to be planned and integrated to provide a coherent service for the community.

Chapter 9

Action to reduce alcohol-related harm must include action at a local level. This will entail co-operation between many different agencies including health authorities, local authorities, police, probation, voluntary agencies, and the Licensing Bench. All these agencies need to meet and develop a common strategy for both prevention of harm and provision of help to those who have already been harmed. Once the strategy has been written it must be implemented.

Examples of local initiatives include work with schools, work with young people and provision of alcohol-free alternatives such as 'alcohol-free pubs'. The workplace is one location where local action can be taken by developing workplace alcohol policies. Local forums (meetings) with the licensing magistrates are another method of stimulating local action. Development of services for ethnic minorities, services for offenders, after care schemes for discharged prisoners, and services for the homeless are other examples of ways in which the local services can be developed to meet local needs.

Chapter 10

A large number of people earn their living making or selling alcoholic drinks and it is important that their interests should be considered. While it is necessary for the public health interest to limit the quantity of alcoholic products which are sold, there are many issues on which health promoters and the industry can make common cause. It is not in the interests of the drinks industry to damage the health of their customers.

Some industry initiatives, such as the Wheelwatch campaign and education campaigns for customers, must be wholeheartedly welcomed. Product labelling is another area where the industry could co-operate with health promoters. Labelling drinks with their strength and selling them in units or simple multiples of a unit would make it easier for customers to monitor their own drinking. Appropriate health warnings on the containers could also be helpful. The development of a wide range of low alcohol or non-alcohol alternatives to alcoholic drinks is another move from industry which has much to recommend it. These products enable the industry to develop their market and increase profits without increasing alcohol consumption.

Advertising is an area of dispute. Though it is alleged that advertising serves only to encourage switching between brands it seems plausible that it also encourages more consumption. Advertising of alcoholic drinks is governed by a voluntary code which require among other things that advertisements should not suggest that alcohol increase sexual attractiveness or use young people to promote the product. The code is widely flouted. There is certainly a need for much closer examination of the effects of advertising on drinking patterns.


Chapter 11

The medical profession has not made the contribution to reducing the risk to public health posed by alcohol which it might have. This state of affairs may be accounted for by inadequate training in medical schools and postgraduate courses.

Alcohol has occupied little time in the medical school curriculum and where it appeared was often discussed in terms of alcoholic stereotypes rather than as a risk factor. Deficient knowledge has been compounded by inappropriate attitudes.

Heavy drinking has traditionally been a feature of medical schools and it is not surprising that too many doctors have themselves become unduly reliant on alcohol as an aid to relaxation and relief of stress. They are then less able to identify and intervene with patients whose drinking patterns threaten their health.

The deficiencies have begun to be remedied in some general practitioner and other training schemes. There is a need to review all medical training to ensure doctors are equipped to recognise alcohol problems at a stage where they are relatively easy to resolve, and to offer appropriate interventions. Doctors have a special responsibility to defend the public health and they must therefore be prepared to set an example of healthy drinking.

## Chapter 12

The purpose of public health medicine is not simply to describe problems but also to take action to reduce those problems. We have therefore made a series of recommendations as to how alcohol-related harm to the public health can be reduced. In this final chapter, we list Government departments and other agencies which ought to take responsibility for implementing the recommendations. We hope that they will be widely debated and then acted upon.

## ▶ Summary

Alcohol used wisely can add to enjoyment of life but increasingly we see evidence that public health is being damaged as a result of alcohol consumption. The damage affects not just an unfortunate minority who drink very heavily, but the whole population.

In the light of this damage to public health we need to review public policy in relation to alcohol. Measures to reduce the harm must include health education so that people really are in a position to make informed choices about their own drinking, reduction of circumstances which pressure people to increase consumption and modification of the environment so as to limit alcohol associated harm.

The response so far from government and the medical profession has been confused and inconsistent. This report presents a series of recommendations which would protect the public health and reduce the present burden of avoidable ill health resulting from unwise consumption of alcohol.

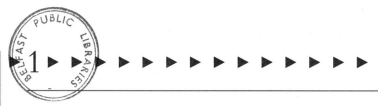

# HOW MUCH DO WE DRINK?

## ▶ A short history of consumption

The art of producing alcoholic beverages by fermentation has been known to virtually every culture, and alcoholic drinks are consumed in a very wide range of societies in the world today.

Alcoholic drinks have been consumed in the British Isles since before records began. Our Celtic ancestors drank mead and ale when they feasted. Roman, Anglo-Saxon, Viking and Norman conquests did not change the widespread consumption of these drinks which continued to be the main beverage of the population until Tudor times. Early in the sixteenth century new brewing techniques which produced a more bitter ale were introduced from the Continent. This drink, known as beer, rapidly replaced meads and less bitter ales as the main drink of the population and has remained popular ever since.

> Hops, Reformation, bays and beer
> Came to England all in one year

Wine drinking was widespread among the wealthy in Roman times when Britain was recognised as a significant wine-producing area. Wines from the Continent were important articles of trade and this trade increased after the Norman Conquest. Wine drinking remained common among the wealthy throughout the Middle Ages. The loss of territory on the Continent and then the dissolution of the monasteries which resulted in the disappearance of British vineyards reduced consumption of wine in Britain. Despite this the wealthy continued to drink wine, especially port.

Prior to the Restoration relatively few spirits were consumed but after this time consumption of brandy and Dutch gin increased. Consumption of spirits was further increased by the

11

introduction of home-produced products and in the early eighteenth century vast quantities of cheap, low-quality spirit were being sold. The notorious sales pitch, 'drunk for one penny, dead drunk for twopence and straw for nothing' dates from this time.

Government always has need of revenue and it was not surprising that the they looked to the flourishing trade in alcohol to provide it. King John introduced a tax on wine imports, and beer duties were first imposed in 1643 to help pay for the Civil War. By the mid-eighteenth century the duties on alcohol were producing a useful source of revenue for government, and Customs and Excise were compiling financial accounts from which it is possible to make fairly reliable estimates of consumption.[1]

These records show that consumption at the start of the eighteenth century was prodigious, equating to more than two pints of beer per man, woman and child per day (or 800 pints per year) (see Figure 1.1). Throughout the eighteenth century it gradually declined to reach a plateau around the year 1800. During the nineteenth century consumption increased in times of prosperity and decreased in times of recession, but there were no sustained changes. The influence of the temperance movement

FIGURE 1.1   *Changes in alcohol consumption over the centuries*

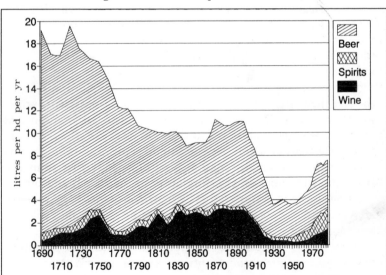

12

and the wakening social conscience of legislators contributed to a fall in consumption beginning about 1900. This was reinforced by controls imposed during the First World War by a Government (see Chapter 5) concerned that productivity in munitions factories was being impaired by drinking. After the war consumption continued to fall and by the mid-1930s recession it was probably at the lowest level it had ever been.

Consumption remained low until the 1950s, when it started to rise as the economy became more prosperous. This trend was reinforced by increasing familiarity with continental drinking habits. Apart from a temporary reduction in consumption associated with the economic depression around 1980, consumption of alcohol has continued to rise and is now close to the level it was at the start of the century. Consumption of beer has remained relatively stable but consumption of wines and, to a lesser extent, spirits have increased significantly (see Figures 5.1 and 5.2 on pages 87 and 88).

## ▶ Alcohol-related problems in the past

Contemporary records indicate that our forebears consumed very large amounts of alcohol. However, death and disease due to alcohol may have been less obvious to them among the mass of death and disease due to other causes at a time when life was nasty, brutish and short. Church authorities found it necessary to order that any priest who got drunk before a service should do three days penance but did not regard alcohol as posing a great threat to the souls of the laity.[2] The first major licensing acts were passed in the reign of Elizabeth I and gave the local justices wide powers to regulate beer and wine sales. Drunkenness was well recognised and whipping or a spell in the stocks was considered appropriate treatment for this condition.

Anxieties about the effect of alcohol on society first seem to have troubled legislators in Georgian times when gin and other spirits had become very cheap. The poor consumed these in vast quantities and the resulting public drunkenness, debauchery, ill-health and alcohol-related crime were too obvious to be ignored. The chairman of one metropolitan Bench warned that, 'excessive drinking of gin and other pernicious spirits was destructive of lives, families and trades'. A little later a committee of the

Middlesex Sessions complained of begging, pilfering and stealing by children of drinking parents.[3] Parliament responded to this outcry by a series of Gin Acts which virtually put the gin sellers out of business.

Concern about alcohol was however very selective. William Hogarth, the artist, at the same time as attacking the evils and misery of Gin Lane lauded the healthy joys of Beer Street. The wickedness of intoxication among the poor was generally preached but intoxication among the gentry seemed acceptable.

As the Industrial Revolution transformed Britain from an agricultural to a post agricultural economy the effects of alcohol on society and especially the poor gave rise to more concern. The contribution of alcohol to neglect of children, wife-beating, debt, loss of trade, and accidents was generally noted. Parliament responded with a series of alehouse and beerhouse acts which placed increasing restrictions on the sale of alcohol. The temperance movement founded in 1832 by Joseph Livesey denounced the obvious evils of excessive drinking and, allied with the non-conformist churches, persuaded a large section of the population not to drink any alcohol.

## ▶ Alcohol in different countries

Alcohol consumption in Britain is rather less than in most European countries (see Figure 1.2). Countries differ not only in the overall amount of alcohol consumed but also in the types of beverage and circumstances in which alcohol is consumed. The United Kingdom, along with Denmark, the Republic of Ireland and Germany is predominantly a beer-drinking culture. In other countries, such as France, Spain and Italy, wine is the predominant drink while in yet other countries such as Sweden and Poland spirits predominate.[4]

Cirrhosis mortality rates, prevalence rates for 'alcoholism', admission rates for 'alcoholic psychoses', mortality from alcohol-related causes, arrests for drunkenness and alcohol-related public order offences, and drink-drive offence rates may all be used as indicators of the frequency of alcohol-related harm in a country. However, poorly defined diagnostic criteria, differences in attitudes to alcohol-related harm, differences in law and

FIGURE 1.2    *Comparison of alcohol consumption in different countries around 1985*

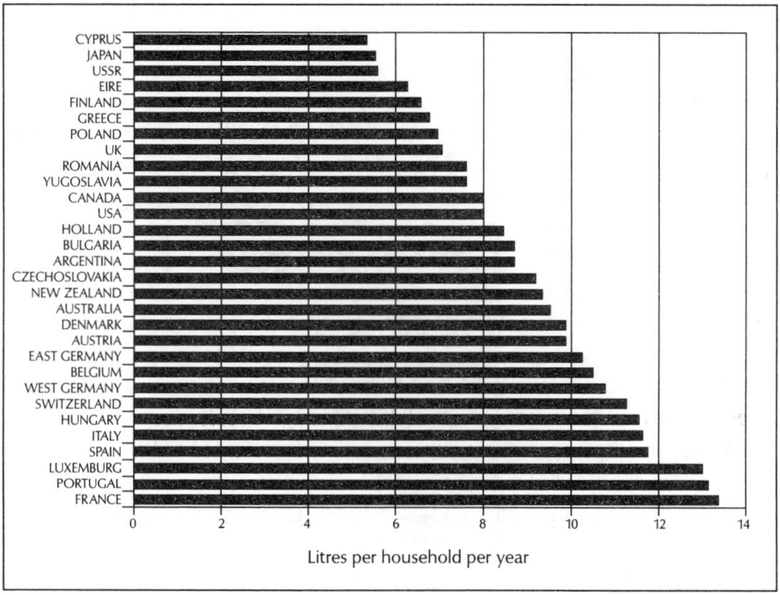

SOURCE    E. Crooks, *Alcohol consumption and taxation* (IFS Report Series No. 34, 1989), Table 2.4

differences in data recording make it very difficult to compare such data between countries.[5,6]

Cirrhosis mortality (see Figure 1.3) shows wide variation between countries. In general, countries with the highest consumption have the highest mortality rates from cirrhosis though there are anomalies. Estimates of prevalence rates for 'alcoholism' have to be treated with extreme caution since it is usually not clear how the term is defined. None the less, the estimates suggest that prevalence rates are higher in countries with high consumption, such as France, Luxemburg and Switzerland.

It is often suggested that in Scandinavian and northern European countries people tend to drink alcohol in situations where drinking is the main activity and to drink in bouts, whereas in Mediterranean wine-drinking countries drinking activity is more likely to be associated with eating and to be

15

FIGURE 1.3    *Cirrhosis mortality rates in different countries (deaths per 100,000)*

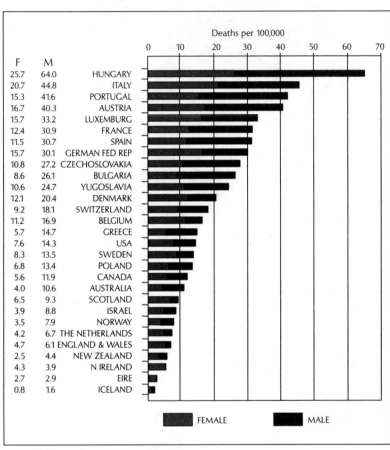

The rates shown are for the most recent year available (1986 or 1987) in all countries except three. The rates are crude rates and make no allowance for difference in age structure of the population.

Note: The black bars representing the male rates start from zero and are not added on top of the female rates.

SOURCE:    *Statistical Yearbook* (World Health Organisation, 1988.)

more evenly spread over time. The northern drinking pattern is reputed to be associated with a high frequency of problems related to acute intoxication and public disorder whereas such problems are suggested to be less common with the Mediterranean drinking pattern. Alcohol-related public disorder offences are certainly a problem in Scandinavian countries[7] and in Poland, but alcohol-related crime and violence may be commoner in countries such as France and Italy[8] than is generally believed.

## ▶ Consumption in Britain

The population of England and Wales in 1987 spent £17 billion on alcohol[9] equivalent to £370 for every adult in Britain. Estimates of consumption come from two sources: Customs and Excise data and population surveys. Excise data covers only the alcohol on which duty has been paid and thus excludes home brewed alcohol, alcohol consumed outside the country and alcohol imported as duty free allowance. Alcohol consumed by overseas visitors and alcohol on which duty is paid but is not drunk has to be set against this. It is also necessary to make assumptions about the alcohol content of the beverages recorded in the excise records. All these factors introduce errors but it is likely that estimates of total consumption based on excise figures are broadly correct.

Population surveys, however, consistently produce figures much lower than excise data. Drinking patterns by age and sex derived from the OPCS 1987 survey[10] are shown in Figure 1.4. It can be calculated from these figures that annual consumption is 4.2 litres of absolute alcohol per head compared to the estimate from excise data of 7.4 litres of absolute alcohol per head. The reasons for this discrepancy are a tendency for people, especially heavy drinkers, to underestimate their own consumption and for higher non-response rates among heavy and problem drinkers. Five per cent of men and 8 per cent of women do not drink alcohol at all and among those aged over sixty-five the figures rise to 10 per cent and 15 per cent respectively.

Differences in drinking patterns can be identified between groups. There are variations between the amount consumed by different social classes (see Figure 1.5). Males drink more than females, especially in the younger age groups, and younger adults

FIGURE 1.4 *Drinking category by age and sex.*

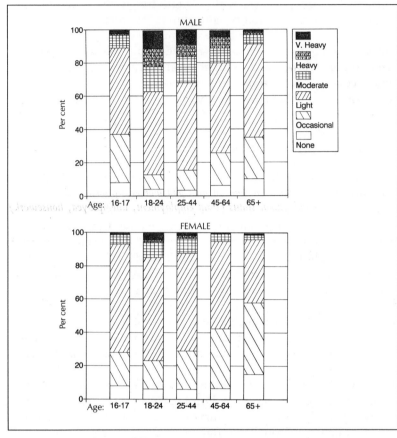

Drinkers are defined as follows:

| | |
|---|---|
| None | No alcohol in last year |
| Occasional | No alcohol in last month |
| Light for males | Less than 22 units per week |
|    "   " females | Less than 15 units per week |
| Moderate for males | 22–35 units |
|    "   " females | 15–25 units |
| Heavy for males | 36–50 units |
|    "   " females | 26–35 units |
| Very heavy for males | More than 50 units per week |
|    "    "   " females | More than 35 units per week |

SOURCE: E. Goddard and C. Ikin, *Drinking in England and Wales in 1987* (OPCS Social Survey division, 1988).

drink more than older adults. Among men there is considerable regional variation in amount consumed but among women no variation is apparent (see Figure 1.6).

Comparison between consecutive surveys (see Figure 1.7) shows that drinking patterns in men have changed little over the past ten years but in women there is a tendency for higher consumption in most ages groups.[11]

FIGURE 1.5    *Consumption level in men and women by social class and employment status (Paid employment, unemployed, housework)*

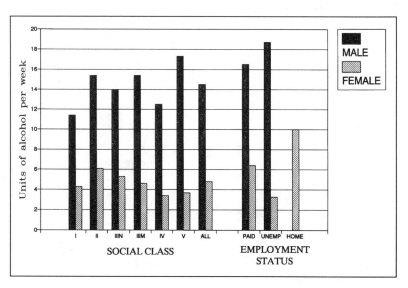

SOURCE:    As Figure 1.4.

FIGURE 1.6  *Mean consumption in units per week for men and women in England and Wales*

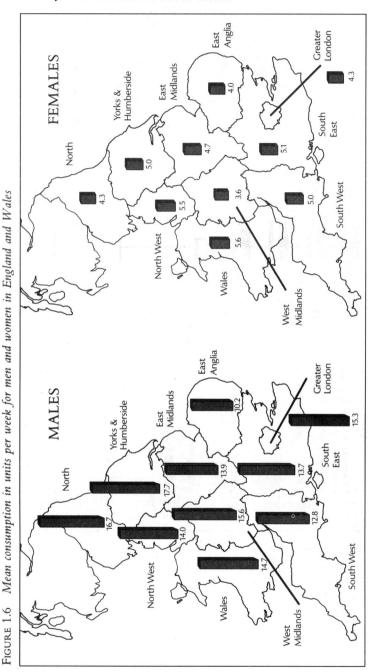

This survey did not cover Northern Ireland or Scotland but surveys in 1980 showed mean consumption (units per week) as follows: England and Wales: men 14.9; women 4.0; Scotland: men 15.2; women 3.4; Northern Ireland: men 6.7; women 1.3.

SOURCE  *As Figure 1.4*

FIGURE 1.7    *Changes in consumption by age and sex between 1978 and 1987*

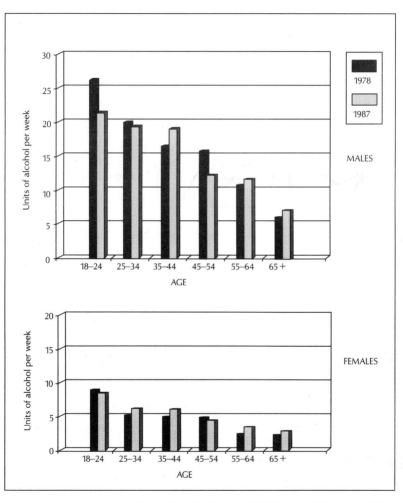

Large surveys were conducted in England and Wales in 1978 and 1987. The results are compared in this figure.

SOURCE    As Figure 1.4

References

1. J. A. Spring and D. H. Buss 'Three centuries of alcohol in the British diet', *Nature*, 270(1977), pp. 567–72.
2. N. Longmate 'Alcohol and the family in history', in J. Orford and J. Harwin (eds) *Alcohol and the family* (London: Croom Helm, 1982).
3. Ibid.
4. R. G. Smart 'Is the post-war drinking binge ending? Cross national trends in per capita alcohol consumption', *British Journal of Addiction*, 84(1989), pp. 743–48.
5. P. Davies and D. Walsh (eds) *Alcohol problems and alcohol control in Europe* (London: Croom Helm, 1983).
6. N. Giesbrecht, M. Cahannes, J. Moskalewicz, E. Osterberg and R. Room (eds) *Consequences of drinking; Trends in alcohol problem statistics in seven countries* (Toronto: Addiction Research Foundation, 1983).
7. P. Davies and D. Walsh, op. cit.
8. Ibid.
9. C.S.O. *Annual abstract of statistics*, No. 25 (London: HMSO, 1989).
10. N. E. Goddard and C. Ikin, *Drinking in England and Wales in 1987* (London: OPCS Social Survey Division, HMSO, 1988)
11. N. Giesbrecht *et al.*, op. cit.

# ▶ 2 ▶ ▶ ▶ ▶ ▶ ▶ ▶ ▶ ▶ ▶ ▶ ▶ ▶ ▶ ▶

# MEDICAL AND PSYCHIATRIC PROBLEMS RELATED TO ALCOHOL USE

## ▶ The benefits of alcohol

It may be surprising to find a section entitled the benefits of alcohol in a report on alcohol and the public health but it is the intention of this report to review the evidence and not to propagandise. However, the very widespread use of alcohol in our society (and the experience of individual members of the working party) suggests that in certain circumstances the use of alcohol increases enjoyment and well-being and contributes to social support networks.

The literature on alcohol contains many examples of problems related to its use and many of them are described in this book, but relatively little attention has been paid to its beneficial effects. Authors often appear to have made a 'presumption against alcohol' and one needs to critically assess whether this is justified in each situation.

Alcohol use is so intimately woven into the fabric of many people's everyday social and psychological functioning that it is very difficult to determine what is and what is not alcohol-related. The evidence is often incomplete and frequently we have no example of an alcohol-free situation with which to make comparisons. Sometimes, as when considering accidents or the workplace, the evidence of alcohol-related harm is overwhelming (see later in this chapter). In other situations, such as the effect on family life, the situation is more complex and there are real if poorly-defined benefits to be set against the harmful effects.

From a public health standpoint we need to accept that there is a balance sheet: the aim should be to minimise the harmful effects of alcohol while fostering the beneficial effects. Strategies have to be not against alcohol but against the harms caused by alcohol. None the less, in many instances a reduction in alcohol consumption will be an essential component of harm reduction.

# ▶ Alcohol–related harm

All sorts of harm to public health is associated with the use of alcohol. Table 2.1 lists some of those harms.

TABLE 2.1   *Alcohol-related harm*

Physical ill-health
Psychological ill-health
Public disorder, violence and other crime
Family disputes, marriage breakup
Child neglect and abuse
Road traffic accidents
Accidents at work and in the home
Fire
Drowning
Employment problems

# ▶ Alcohol–related disease

The list of diseases which can be caused by alcohol is long and covers virtually every medical speciality (see Table 2.2). Two of these conditions, cancer and stroke (cerebrovascular accident), are picked out for discussion here because of their great importance from a public viewpoint. They are among the commonest causes of death in the United Kingdom: in order of frequency these causes are heart disease, cancer, respiratory disease and stroke. Other alcohol–related diseases are discussed in more detail in the report of the Royal College of Physicians.[1]

▶ Alcohol and cancer

If it can be shown that people who drink alcohol have a higher risk of getting a particular cancer, alcohol and that cancer are said to be associated, but just because two things are associated does not prove that one causes the other. However, if for any cancer the association with alcohol is strong and consistent and if there is other supporting evidence, then it is reasonable to conclude that the association is causal and that alcohol is a contributory cause for that cancer.

The relation between alcohol and cancer in humans has recently been examined in an extensive review[2] which concluded with the words 'alcoholic beverages are carcinogenic to humans'. It has been estimated that 3 per cent of all cancers might be attributable to alcohol.[3]

Other studies have consistently shown that the risk of cancers of the oral cavity and pharynx in heavy drinkers was more than double that in non-drinkers and the risk increased as daily intake of alcohol increased. Similarly, nearly all epidemiological studies of cancer of the larynx and cancer of the oesophagus show increased risks in heavy drinkers compared to non-drinkers. It is sometimes difficult to distinguish the effects of smoking and drinking in studies of this sort but when smoking is taken into account, the association with alcohol is still clearly present. The effects of alcohol seem to be synergistic with those of smoking so that the increased risk associated with alcohol is even greater in smokers than in non-smokers.[4] Primary cancer of the liver can also be caused by alcohol consumption.

Three case control studies have shown an association between rectal cancer and consumption of beer (but not other alcoholic beverages). However, several other studies did not support this observation and the data can be called no more than suggestive. A particular association of cancer with beer would not be surprising since beer contains appreciable levels of N-nitrosoamines,[5] though the levels produced by modern brewing techniques are lower than those produced by more traditional methods.

Some studies have suggested an association of cancer of the breast and drinking.[6,7] Even consumption of 14 units per week may be associated with increased risk.[8] There are many other risk factors which might confound this association, so conclusions must be guarded at present. The evidence on alcohol and breast

TABLE 2.2   *Physical conditions which may be associated with alcohol consumption*

---

*Nervous system*
Acute intoxication, blackouts
Wernicke's encephalopathy, Korsakoffs syndrome, cerebellar degeneration, dementia
Strokes, subarachnoid haemorrhage, subdural haematoma
Withdrawal symptoms, tremor, hallucinations, fits
Peripheral neuropathy

*Gastrointestinal*
Liver: fatty change, alcoholic hepatitis, cirrhosis
Oesophagus: reflux oesophagitis, oesophageal tears, oesophageal varices
Stomach: gastritis, aggravation of peptic ulcers
Diarrhoea and malabsorption
Pancreatitis

*Heart and circulation*
Abnormal rhythms, cardiomyopathy
High blood pressure

*Respiratory system*
Pneumonia from inhaled vomit
Fractured ribs

*Cancer*
Liver, oesophagus, larynx, pharynx, ?breast

*Reproductive system*
*Men*: loss of libido, impotency, shrinkage of genitalia, reduced sperm formation, infertility
*Women*: Sexual difficulties, menstrual irregularities, shrinkage of breasts and genitalia
Foetal alcohol syndrome

*Accidents, falls and injuries*
Head injuries
Suicide
Other injuries

*Endocrine system and nutrition*
Over-production of adrenal hormones
Thyrotoxicosis-like state
Hypoglycaemia
Obesity

*Interactions with medication*

---

cancer is difficult to interpret and some authorities do not accept that alcohol is a cause of breast cancer.[9, 10] Any elevation of risk with alcohol is likely to be modest (25–50 per cent) but would be important since cancer of the breast is the commonest cancer in women.

There have been suggestions that many other types of cancer are associated with alcohol, but where there is sufficient evidence to form a judgement they appear unlikely to be causally related to cancer.

## ▶ Alcohol and stroke

Stroke is a major public health problem both as a cause of death and as a cause of disabling disease. Heavy drinking appears to increase the risk of strokes in men. A study of men admitted to hospital in Birmingham with strokes suggested that the risk was four times greater in those who drank thirty or more units per week compared to non-drinkers.[11] Long-term population studies in other parts of the world also suggest an association. There is little information on women but a recent study from Boston, USA, found an increased risk of haemorrhagic strokes with drinking but a decreased risk of other types of stroke.[12]

## ▶ Alcohol-related mortality

Heavy drinkers have long been recognised to have a greatly increased risk of dying prematurely. One large study showed that men who had alcohol problems sufficiently severe to warrant admission to a mental hospital had a greatly increased mortality (see Figure 2.1).[13] The chief causes of increased mortality are suicides, accidents, respiratory infections, strokes and cancer. Alcohol as a causal factor is mentioned on very few death certificates and cirrhosis, though occurring far more often in heavy drinkers than in the general population, is still a relatively uncommon cause of death.

Studies of those with severe alcohol problems are illuminating in telling us possible causes of death but say little about the numbers of deaths attributable to alcohol consumption in the population. Several large population studies allow us to relate

FIGURE 2.1   *Causes of death in male 'alcoholics'*

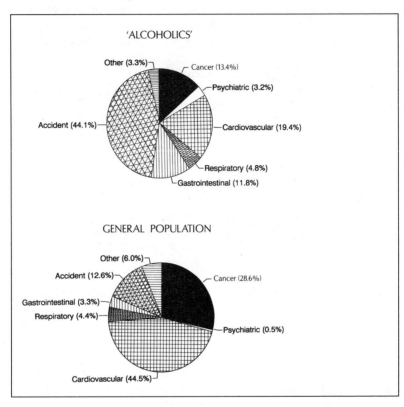

The calculated age-adjusted causes of death from the data in Adelstein and White (1976) are compared with those of the general population (1986).

Note that the mortality rate in the 'alcoholics' is three and a half times greater than that in the general population.

'Alcoholics' were defined as those discharged from a mental hospital with a primary diagnosis of alcoholic psychosis.

alcohol consumption to subsequent mortality. Nearly all these studies show a U-shaped curve with the lowest mortality in those who consume small amounts and higher mortality both in abstainers and in heavy drinkers.[14] Figure 2.2 shows data from one British study[15] which illustrates this relationship.

FIGURE 2.2    *Death rates from cardiovascular and non-cardiovascular causes in different categories of drinker from the British Regional Heart survey.*

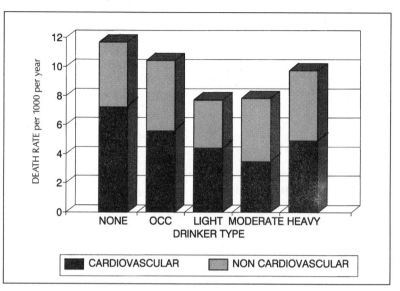

None = total abstainer, Occ (occasional), Light, Moderate and Heavy drinker respectively < 1, 1–15, 16–42 and > 42 units per week.

SOURCE    Figure – A. G. Shaper, G. Wannamathee and M. Walker, 'Alcohol and Mortality in British men: Explaining the U shaped curve', *The Lancet*, ii(1988) pp. 1267–73.

The slight excess mortality in abstainers has been the subject of much debate. It is in part explained by the observation that people who are ill tend to become abstainers[16] (see also Chapter 8 page 137) but this may not be the entire explanation. It is possible that small amounts of alcohol might confer some protection against heart disease since it raises HDL (high density lipoprotein) cholesterol[17] though it is not clear whether the HDL fraction affected protects the heart.[18] It is also certain that alcohol contributes to hypertension (high blood pressure)[19] and this would counteract any beneficial effect on lipids (fats) in the bloodstream. The evidence does not justify any suggestion that abstainers would benefit their health if they started to consume alcohol.

Estimates of the deaths attributable to alcohol consumption in England and Wales vary from 5000 to 40,000. P. Anderson[20] arrived at a figure of 28,000 deaths attributable to alcohol. He did this by multiplying the numbers of people drinking at different levels in the population of England and Wales by the death rates seen in people drinking at those levels taken from a study in the USA.[21] This is equivalent to a loss of 560,000 life years, a figure which is much greater than the 185,000 life years upper estimate arrived at by McDonnell and Maynard.[22]

## ▶ Hospital workload

Many studies have shown that heavy drinkers are heavy users of hospital services. Repeated studies[23, 24, 25, 26, 27, 28] have shown that between 12 and 27 per cent of men admitted to general medical wards have features indicative of problem drinking. The proportion of women with these features is less but still appreciable. Heavy drinkers are particularly likely to have taken overdoses.

Heavy drinking is also common in patients attending accident and emergency departments. A breath alcohol meter was used to assess recent consumption in patients attending an Edinburgh accident and emergency department in the evening and night[29] and showed that a high proportion had been drinking (see Figure 2.3). Another study in Hull[30] showed that 14 per cent of all accident and emergency attendances were alcohol-related but this figure rose to 24 per cent between 8.00 pm and midnight and 46 per cent between midnight and 6.00 am Studies from elsewhere[31, 32] confirm the frequency of high levels of breath alcohol in those attending accident and emergency departments.

## ▶ General practice workload

Patients with alcohol problems consult their general practitioners nearly twice as often as the average patient,[33] the most common problems being gastrointestinal, psychiatric and accidents. A typical general practitioner will have about 2000 patients on his or her list, which could be expected to include about 40 patients who could be designated as problem drinkers and a further 100

FIGURE 2.3   *Proportion of casualty attenders having positive breath test for alcohol by diagnostic group.*

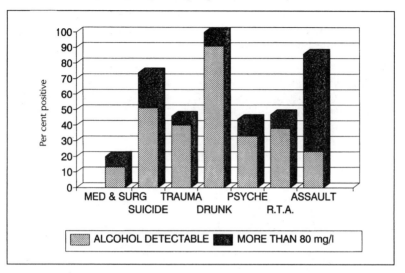

Med & Surg = General Medical and Surgical Conditions;
Psyche = Psychiatric; R.T.A. = Road Traffic Accidents

SOURCE   Holt *et al.*, 'Alcohol and the emergency service patient', *British Medical Journal*, 281(1980) pp. 638–40.

who are at high risk of developing problems because they are heavy drinkers yet the general practitioner is likely to be unaware of the alcohol problem in more than half of the affected patients. These estimates have been confirmed by surveys.[34] Patients with alcohol-related problems, because of their large numbers and their increased use of services, make a very significant contribution to the general practitioner's workload.

The methodology of virtually all the studies cited, whether in hospital or general practice, could be criticised: some studies failed to define what was meant by an alcohol-related problem; others reported the frequency of heavy or problem drinkers in populations of patients but did not use control groups of non-patients or explain whether the illness was causally related to their drinking.[35] There is a need for more rigorous studies to quantify the excess risk of ill-health attributable to alcohol use.

Despite these weaknesses, the existing studies of hospital admissions, casualty attendances and general practice studies all tell the same story. Alcohol-related problems are common, cause extra work in all parts of the health service and load a considerable burden of avoidable ill-health on the community.

---

### Recommendation No. 1

It is recommended that large-scale longitudinal studies should include data on alcohol consumption so that the mortality and morbidity risk associated with different consumption levels in this country can be defined.

---

### Recommendation No. 2

It is recommended that special surveys should be undertaken in hospitals and general practice so that the extra workload attributable to alcohol use can be identified.

---

## ▶ Alcohol in pregnancy

So far we have discussed the effect of alcohol on the health of the individual consuming it, but an unborn child can also be affected by alcohol consumed by its mother. Some children born to mothers with severe alcohol problems were noted to have a syndrome characterised by growth retardation, neurological abnormalities and facial malformations (the foetal alcohol syndrome).[36, 37] Later it became apparent that the same features were occasionally found in children born to mothers who had drunk relatively modest amounts in pregnancy. The risk to the foetus increases as the mother's alcohol consumption increases but it is not clear whether there is a safe limit for alcohol intake in pregnancy below which there is no risk. It is likely that there may be critical stages in the development of the embryo when it is especially vulnerable to alcohol.

A large American study[38] showed no difference in birth weight between children born to mothers who abstained totally during pregnancy and those born to mothers who drank less than one unit per day during pregnancy. While mothers would be well advised to drink very little while pregnant there is little evidence to suggest that total abstinence throughout pregnancy is necessary.

## ▶ Unwanted pregnancy

Control of their own fertility should be one of the benefits of modern life for women but unwanted pregnancies continue to occur. These pregnancies may cause damage to the health of the mother and increased risk to the health of the child if it is born. The social and cultural influences which lead people to risk unwanted pregnancies are complex but alcohol is implicated especially in the young. Among fourteen-year-olds, 35 per cent of boys and 44 per cent of girls reported [39] that they had drunk so much that they could not remember what happened in the preceding night at least once in the past three months. In many cases one of the events forgotten may have been unprotected intercourse, which is much more likely to occur after drinking.

## ▶ Alcohol and AIDS

A major threat to public health is posed by the new disease of AIDS (Acquired Immune Deficiency Syndrome) which is caused by the HIV (Human Immunodeficiency Virus) virus. Though most current cases in the United Kingdom have been transmitted through homosexual intercourse or less frequently through intravenous drug use, transmission through heterosexual intercourse is likely to become much more frequent in the future. The behaviours which place individuals at risk are unprotected intercourse and intercourse with a large number of different partners. As discussed in the preceding section, alcohol use and intoxication increase the likelihood of a young person engaging in these risky types of behaviour.[40] Alcohol also affects the immune system[41] and may therefore increase the risk that an individual becomes HIV positive when exposed to the virus. It is impossible to quantify the contribution of alcohol to the spread of AIDS but it clearly plays a part in some cases.

# ▶ Psychological effects of alcohol

The psychological effects of alcohol can be divided into *immediate*, such as intoxication; *delayed*, such as hangover; and *long-term*, such as dementia. The immediate effects are due to the pharmacological actions of alcohol while the delayed and long-term effects can be either organic or functional. An organic effect or state is one which is based on structural damage to the brain while a functional effect or state is one which apparently does not involve structural damage to the brain.

The psychological effects of alcohol use are learned and therefore somewhat culture specific. How people feel and behave after drinking alcohol is governed by a complex interaction of their expectations of its effect, their psychological and physical state at the time of drinking and the social setting in which drinking takes place.

# ▶ Intoxication

Intoxication is a great mimic and a much more complex state than is implied by the old notion of loss of inhibitions resulting from 'suppression of higher centres'. Generally, mild intoxication leads to increased self esteem, increased perceived personal power and probably a feeling of relaxation. This package of increased confidence and relaxation may enhance sociability and facilitate social interaction.

Other aspects of intoxication are less benign. Expectations of alcohol's action are learnt and, in Western cultures, we tend to learn that alcohol does indeed remove inhibitions and therefore increases the probability of violence. In Britain, release of aggressiveness, inclinations to sexually demanding, dominant behaviour and 'boisterous' petty theft and criminal damage are all seen as part of the alcohol 'intoxication package'.[42]

This expectation is far from universal and anthropologists have drawn our attention to other cultures where intoxication has very different connotations, including, in one example, no mood effect at all; only clumsiness.[43]

## ▶ Alcohol amnesia

Alcohol amnesias or 'blackouts' are very common. Around a quarter of all men have had one.[44] They are described as 'an alcohol-related inability to remember an ordinarily memorable event'. They are reported more commonly by people who come to the doctor with alcohol problems and are said to be organically based rather than functional mental states. However, the tendency of these amnestic attacks to occur before some event that would be well worth forgetting, such as domestic violence, committing a criminal act or failing sexually suggests that they may not be entirely organic. There is a clear similarity between this transient state and the permanent condition known as Korsakoff's Amnestic State in which there is structural brain damage (see page 37).

## ▶ Delayed effects of alcohol

It is important to remember that the majority of episodes of alcohol use do not have delayed effects of note, either positive or negative. However, there are acute (reversible) consequences which occur in some people after certain drinking occasions.

## ▶ Hangover

Like intoxication, a hangover is a complex state and again its presentation is to some extent culturally determined. It is said that that much cited tribe the Camba of South America, who were prodigious bout drinkers, did not suffer from hangover (or, indeed from other withdrawal states) because the tribe's cultural beliefs did not recognise the phenomenon.[45] In the West, we do recognise the hangover and it would appear to comprise four components, a direct effect of alcohol on the gut, (giving rise to anorexia (lack of appetite), nausea and diarrhoea); dehydration; positional alcohol nystagmus (involuntary jerky movements of the eyes); and minor withdrawal phenomena.

Along with these four clear effects, there tend to be mental changes characterised by guilt, misery and a (usually unsustained) resolve never to get into that state again.[46] It is notable that some people with hangovers have not made the link between their mood state and the hangover: they do not know that last night's drinking was the cause of this morning's misery.

## ▶ Withdrawal phenomena

The notion that hangover has as one of its components withdrawal phenomena is relatively new and perhaps still contentious, but it makes sense because withdrawal states are now seen as being on a continuum ranging from trivial to very severe. The features of withdrawal may include eating disturbance, tremor, paroxysmal sweats, clouding of senses, hallucinations, impaired quality of contact, agitation, sleep disturbance, raised temperature, elevated pulse rate and convulsions. One or more of these features can be experienced in greater or lesser degrees by hangover sufferers. They are also components of a number of functional psychiatric disorders such as anxiety states and agitated depression.

## ▶ Chronic organic consequences of alcohol use

The majority of drinkers do not suffer long term psychological problems as a result of their drinking careers. However, there are some states which are clearly related to alcohol use, and these are discussed below.

### Psychological deficits (impairment)

Psychological impairment associated with alcohol range from minor to severe. Minor degrees of impairment, which are often noted in young heavy drinkers, involve loss of dexterity and co-ordination, and loss of clear thinking, leading to a slowness in problem-solving. At the other end of the scale, alcohol-induced dementia can occur, producing a condition which, apart from the history of heavy alcohol use, is clinically indistinguishable from Alzheimer's disease.[47]

## Paranoid states

Paranoid states are states characterised by delusions. Alcohol-associated paranoid states can be classified into states without psychological impairment, states with marginal impairment and states with marked impairment. Patients with paranoid states without impairment may be difficult to detect. They often first come to notice having accused innocent bystanders (in, say, a public house) of talking about them behind their backs. Paranoid states with marked psychological impairment are rather easier to detect. Those affected are clearly impaired and fail to lay down or recall new memory traces so that they might accuse others of stealing money from them because they have no recall of having already spent it, possibly on alcohol. The psychological impairment is made worse by intoxication.

## Korsakoff's Psychosis or Korsakoff's Amnestic State

Korsakoff's amnestic state is characterised by disorientation, a loss of recent memory and a tendency to confabulation (inventing stories to fill memory gaps) in alert, responsive people with no clouding of consciousness.[48] The main feature of the state is the inability to lay down, or arguably retrieve, new memory traces.

## ▶ Functional disorders related to alcohol use

Alcohol use is a major cause of the organic states described in the preceding sections and if alcohol had not been ingested, they would not have occurred. The situation with regard to the functional states is more equivocal. Functional states can, and frequently do, occur without alcohol being present but their presentation may be coloured by alcohol if the patient also drinks. Also, people with alcohol problems often suffer from functional psychiatric disorders as well. People experiencing alcohol withdrawal may complain of insomnia, agitation and hallucinatory states. Even in the absence of recent drinking, former heavy drinkers commonly demonstrate depression, suicidal intent, sexual problems and self neglect.

Alcohol may be implicated in all of the functional disorders. Further, there are a number of people with psychiatric problems who use alcohol as a method of self-medication to deal with their distress. Alcohol is not a good medication for such problems and when it is used in the self-management of functional states such as depression, can become a problem in its own right. Some recent evidence suggests that if someone takes to drinking alcohol as a way of dealing with a primary mood disorder then the primary disorder often becomes secondary to the problems of alcohol use.[49]

In the neuroses, and particularly in phobic and anxiety states, a vicious circle between the disorder and chronic alcohol use is often established. It is striking how often the process of detoxification removes the phobic symptoms along with the signs of alcohol toxicity.[50]

The relationship between alcohol and 'personality disorders' is a definitional minefield which will not be discussed here. Suffice it to say that in many studies, 'personality disorders' are over-represented in clients presenting themselves to alcohol services, and problematic alcohol use is reputed to occur more frequently among people who are said to have personality problems. Problems related to alcohol use and 'personality disorders' are certainly commonly associated but it is impossible to be sure whether one condition predisposes to the other.

## ▶ Accidents, fire and drowning

Accidents are the commonest cause of death in young adults and must be considered a major public health problem. Here too alcohol is implicated. It has already been noted that a large number of those attending casualty departments with accidental injuries have been drinking, and coroners' files also suggest that alcohol is frequently associated with fatal accidents. The contribution of alcohol to accidents at work are discussed in Chapter 3. Alcohol is clearly a major contributory factor to road traffic accidents, which are discussed in Chapter 7.

It is difficult to determine the number of fires where alcohol is involved, though intoxication is likely to increase the chances of starting a fire accidentally and then reduce the chances of escaping from that fire. The Strathclyde Fire Service estimated that 66 per cent of all fire deaths in their area were alcohol-related.[51] The best statistics available on drownings[52] suggest that in recent years 20 per cent of drownings were alcohol-related, however it is accepted that the figures are incomplete and the true number may be even higher.

## References

1. Royal College of Physicians, *A great and growing evil. The medical consequences of alcohol abuse* (London: Tavistock, 1986).
2. World Health Organisation/International Agency for Research on Cancer, 'Alcohol drinking', *IARC Monographs on the evaluation of carcinogenic risks to humans*, Vol. 44 (Lyon, IARC, 1988).
3. R. Doll and R. Peto, *The cause of human cancer*, (Oxford University Press, 1981).
4. A. J. Tuyns, J. Esteve, L. Raymond *et al.*, 'Cancer of the larynx/hypopharynx, tobacco and alcohol', *International Journal of Cancer*, 41(1988), pp. 483–91.
5. T. Wainwright, 'Nitrosamines in malt and beer', *Journal of Institute of Brewers*, 92(1986), pp. 73–80.
6. A. Schatzkin, Y. Jones, R. H. Hoover, P. R. Taylor, L. A. Brinton *et al.*, 'Alcohol consumption and breast cancer in the epidemiologic follow-up of the first National Health and Nutrition Examination Survey', *New England Journal of Medicine*, 316(1987), pp. 1169–73.
7. W. C. Willett, M. J. Stampfer, G. A. Colditz, B. A. Rosner and C. H. Hennekens, 'Moderate alcohol consumption and the risk of breast cancer', *New England Journal of Medicine*, 316(1987), pp. 1174–79.
8. Ibid.
9. WHO/IARC Monographs, op. cit.
10. N. Mantel, 'An analysis of two recent reports in the New England Journal of Medicine associating breast cancer in women with moderate alcohol consumption', *Preventive Medicine*, 17(1988), pp. 672–5.
11. J. S. Gill, A. V. Zezulka, M. J. Shipley, S. K. Gill and D. G. Beevers, 'Stroke and alcohol consumption', *New England Journal of Medicine*, 315(1986), pp. 1041–46.
12. M. J. Stampfer, G. A. Colditz, W. C. Willett, F. E. Speizer and C. H. Hennekens, 'A prospective study of moderate alcohol consumption and the risk of coronary disease and stroke in women', *New England Journal of Medicine*, 319(1988), pp. 267–73.
13. A. Adelstein and G. White, 'Alcoholism and mortality', *Population Trends*, 6(1976), pp. 7–13.

14. M. G. Marmot, 'Alcohol and Coronary Heart disease', *International Journal of Epidemiology*, 13(1984), pp. 160–7.
15. M. G. Marmot, G. Rose, M. J. Shipley and B. J. Thomas, 'Alcohol and Mortality', *Lancet* i, 1981, pp. 1159–61.
16. G. Wannamethee and A. G. Shaper, 'Men who do not drink: A report from the British Regional Heart study', *International Journal of Epidemiology*, 17(1988), pp. 307–16.
17. J. Thornton, C. Symes and K. Heaton, 'Moderate alcohol intake reduces bile cholesterol saturation and raises HDL cholesterol', *Lancet*, ii(1983), pp. 819–22.
18. R. D. Moore and T. A. Pearson, 'Moderate alcohol consumption and coronary artery disease', *Medicine*, 86(1986), pp. 243–67.
19. J. F. Potter, L. T. Bannan and D. G. Beevers, 'Alcohol and Hypertension', *British Journal of Addiction*, 79(1984), pp. 365–72.
20. P. Anderson, 'Excess mortality associated with alcohol consumption', *British Medical Journal*, 297(1988), pp. 824–6.
21. A. L. Klatsky, G. D. Friedman, A. B. Siegelaub, 'Alcohol and mortality: a ten year Kaiser-Permanente experience', *Annals of Internal Medicine*, 95(1981), pp. 139–45.
22. R. McDonnell and A. Maynard, 'Estimation of life years lost from alcohol-related premature death', *Alcohol and alcoholism*, 20(1985), pp. 435–43.
23. C. M. B. Jarman and J. M. Kellett, 'Alcoholism in the general hospital', *British Medical Journal*, ii(1979), pp. 469–72.
24. I. G. Barrison, L. Viola, J. Mumford, R. M. Murray, M. Gordon and I. M. Murray-Lyon, 'Detecting excessive drinking among admissions to a general hospital', *Health Trends*, 14(1982), pp. 80–3.
25. A. G. Jariwalla, P. H. Adams and B. D. Hore, 'Alcohol and acute admissions to hospital', *Health Trends*, 11(1979), pp. 95–7.
26. G. Lloyd, J. Chick, E. Crombie and S. Anderson, 'Problem drinkers in medical wards: consumption patterns and disabilities in newly identified male cases', *British Journal of Addiction*, 81(1986), pp. 789–95.
27. C. L. Taylor, P. Kilbane, N. Passmore and R. Davies, 'Prospective study of alcohol-related admissions in an inner city hospital', *Lancet*, ii(1986), pp. 265–7.
28. S. P. Lockhart, Y. H. Carter, A. M. Straffen, K. K. Pang, J. McLoughlin and J. H. Baron, 'Detection of alcohol consumption as a cause of emergency general medical admissions', *Journal of the Royal Society of Medicine*, 79(1986), pp. 132–6.
29. S. Holt, I. C. Stewart, J. M. J. Dixon, R. A. Elton, T. V. Taylor and K. Little, 'Alcohol and the emergency service patient', *British Medical Journal*, 281(1980), pp. 638–40.

30. M. Backhouse, Qurevitvh T. and Silver V., 'Problem drinkers and the statutory services', *Accident and Emergency*, vol.1 (Hull: Addiction Research Centre, 1986).

31. M. E. Walsh and D. A. D. MacLeod, 'Breath alcohol analysis in the accident and emergency department', *Injury*, 15(1980) pp. 62–6.

32. D. W. Yates, J. M. Hadfield and K. Peters, 'Alcohol consumption of patients attending two accident and emergency departments in North West England', *Journal of Royal Society of Medicine*, 80(1986) pp. 486–9.

33. I. C. Buchan, E. G. Buckley, G. L. S. Deacon, R. Irvine and R. Ryan, 'Problem drinkers and their problems', *Journal of the Royal College of General Practitioners*, 31(1983) pp. 151–3.

34. S. M. Wiseman, S. N. McCarthy and M. C. Mitcheson, 'Assessment of drinking patterns in general practice', *Journal of the Royal College of General Practitioners*, 80(1987) pp. 407–8.

35. I. D. McIntosh, 'Alcohol-related disabilities in general hospital practice: a critical assessment of the evidence', *International Journal of Addictions*, 17(1982) pp. 609–39.

36. J. O. Beattie, 'Alcohol, Pregnancy and the fetus', in G. Chamberlain (ed.) *Contemporary Obstetrics and Gynaecology* (London: Butterworths, 1988).

37. H. L. Rosett and L. Weiner, *Alcohol and the fetus* (Oxford and New York: Oxford University Press, 1984).

38. J. L. Mills, B. I. Graubard, E. E. Harley, E. E. Rhoads and H. W. Berendes, 'Maternal alcohol consumption and birth weight. How much drinking during pregnancy is safe?', *Journal of American Medical Association*, 252(1986) pp. 1875–9.

39. A. Marsh, J. Dobbs and A. White, *Adolescent drinking* (London: OPCS Social Survey Division, HMSO, 1986).

40. L. Siegel, 'AIDS: Relationship to alcohol and other drugs', *Journal of Substance Abuse Treatment*, 3(1986) pp. 271–4.

41. R. R. MacGregor , 'Alcohol and Drugs as Co-factors for AIDS', *Advances in alcohol and substrate abuse*, 7(1987) pp. 47–71.

42. T. Myers, 'Alcohol and Violence: Self reported Alcohol consumption among violent and non-violent male prisoners', in N. Krasner, J. S. Madden and R. J. Walker (eds), *Alcohol-related problems. Room for manoeuvre* (Chichester and New York: John Wiley, 1984).

43. C. MacAndrew and R. B. Edgerton, *Drunken Comportment. A social explanation* (London: Nelson, 1970).

44. D. Cahalan and R. Room, *Problem drinking among American men* (New Jersey: Rutgers University, 1974).

45. C. McAndrew and R. B. Edgerton, *Drunken Comportment*, op. cit.

41

46. R. C. Gunn, 'Hangovers and attitudes towards drinking', *Quarterly Journal of Studies on Alcohol*, 34(1973) pp. 194–8.
47. R. E. Tarter, N. Buonopane, H. McBride and D. V. Schneider, 'Differentiation of Alcoholics', *Archives of General Psychiatry*, 34(1977) pp. 761–8.
48. M. Victor, R. C. Adams and G. H. Collins, *The Wernicke-Korsakoff Syndrome* (Oxford: Blackwell, 1971).
49. K. O'Sullivan, C. Rynne, J. Miller, S. O'Sullivan, V. Fitzpatrick, M. Hux, J. Cooney and A. Clare, 'A follow up study on alcoholics with and without co-existing affective disorder', *British Journal of Psychiatry*, 152(1988) pp. 813–19.
50. T. Stockwell, P. Smail, R. Hodgson and S. Cater, 'Alcohol dependence and phobic anxiety states II: A retrospective study', *British Journal of Psychiatry*, 144(1984) pp. 58–63.
51. P. Tether and L. Harrison, 'Alcohol-related fires and drownings', *British Journal of Addiction*, 81(1986) pp. 425–31.
52. Ibid.

# ALCOHOL AND HARM TO THE COMMUNITY

## ▶ Alcohol and crime

Many people believe that alcohol consumption leads to crime and that heavy drinkers are more likely to engage in criminal activity. While casual experience supports this belief the evidence for it needs to be critically examined.

Criminal activity is often preceded by drinking. A study of crime in a seaside resort[1] showed that a very high percentage of those arrested for any criminal offence had been drinking prior to committing the offence. N. Heather[2] interviewed young offenders in Scotland and found that 63 per cent reported drinking before the offence. Another study of burglary[3] showed that one third of offenders regularly drank before burgling.

Offenders are frequently reported to be heavy drinkers. Heather[4] classified 15 per cent of his sample of young offenders as physically dependent on alcohol and a further 48 per cent as psychologically dependent or showing prodromal (premonitory) signs of such dependency.

Alcohol is often suspected to be particularly associated with violent crime. A classic study by Gilles[5] of murder in West Scotland found that 58 per cent of male murderers and 30 per cent of female murderers were intoxicated at the time they committed the crime, as were 52 per cent of male victims and 32 per cent of female victims. Other studies have variously estimated the percentage of murderers who were intoxicated at 20–70 per cent.[6] Similarly, studies of those arrested for assault give estimates of 15–80 per cent as the proportion of offenders who had been drinking immediately prior to committing the offence.

However, it is difficult to be sure that violent crime is especially associated with alcohol and one study[7] which compared violent-crime offenders with non-violent-crime offenders in a Scottish prison found no difference in their drinking behaviour.

The foregoing discussion leaves no doubt that alcohol is frequently associated with crime but it does not necessarily demonstrate that alcohol causes crime. Another possible explanation for the association is that the personal characteristics or cultural backgrounds which lead to heavy drinking also lead to criminal behaviour. When asked about the reasons for their criminal activity, many offenders did not see their drinking as a cause of their criminal behaviour.[8] Certainly alcohol is directly involved in causing some crimes but it is very difficult to establish whether this is true for a tiny fraction or a sizeable proportion of all criminal activity.

*Recommendation No. 3*

It is recommended that data on the drinking behaviour of offenders should be compared to that of appropriate control populations in order to establish the strength of the association between alcohol and crime. Furthermore, the events leading up to the offences should be explored with a view to clarifying the relationship of alcohol consumption to criminal behaviour.

## ▶ Drunkenness offences

Intoxication is not viewed as an extenuating circumstance and routine statistics do not record whether a crime was associated with alcohol. There are however a series of offences where intoxication is the principle component, such as being drunk in a public place (see Figure 3.1). Records of convictions for these offences are notoriously inaccurate indicators of their frequency because police operational policies vary between forces and over time. Persons breaching these laws may simply be moved on in one area, cautioned in another and charged in a third.

The recently coined term 'lager lout' refers to young people who drink large quantities of alcohol and then engage in aggressive and destructive behaviour. The appearance of a new

FIGURE 3.1    *Findings of guilt (cautions and convictions) for drunkenness, 1961–87*

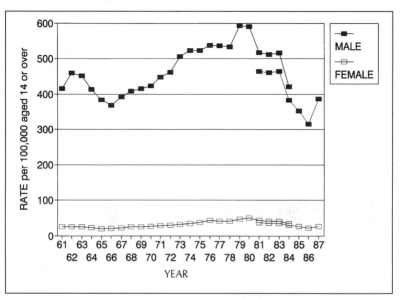

The way in which data are collected was changed in 1981. Prior to 1981 the figures given are for offences (shown by solid line). After that the figures given are for occasions (shown by dashed line), that is where one person was convicted of two offences on the same occasion prior to 1981 they were counted twice but after that year they were counted only once. For the years 1981–84 both types of data are shown to allow comparison.

SOURCE    After 1980, *Offences of Drunkenness in England and Wales*, Home Office Statistical Bulletins. Prior to 1981, *Criminal Statistics Series*, HMSO Command Papers (London, HMSO).

phrase in the language is evidence of public concern and popular belief that alcohol is causally connected with antisocial behaviour.

## ▶ Family disputes and social problems

Heavy drinking can stress a family in many ways. Spending on alcohol and reduced earnings due to the results of drinking alcohol may restrict the family budget, long hours spent drinking outside the home may make the family feel neglected, and intoxicated behaviour may repel or embarrass family members, isolating them from their friends and neighbours. The drinking member of the family may fail to adopt expected roles as parent or spouse and the family may be forced into all sorts of coping strategies. It is not surprising that drinking behaviour is frequently implicated in family breakdown.

Figure 3.2 is taken from the General Household Survey and shows how separated and divorced men tend to drink much more heavily than married or single men. These figures could be explained by increased drinking after the breakdown of marriage but common experience suggests that many were heavy drinkers before the breakdown. The families of drinkers have been noted to have a large number of problems in general practice studies.[9] Violence in marriage is one cause of marital breakdown and alcohol is often mentioned by a 'battered' wife as a factor in their husbands behaviour.[10, 11]

FIGURE 3.2   *Categories of drinker by marital state (men aged 25–44)*

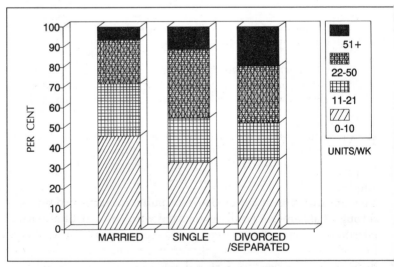

The divorced/separated category also includes widowers, but in this age-band widowers will be a very small minority.

SOURCE   *General Household Survey 1986 Supplement A – Drinking.* (OPCS, 1989).

46

The effect of alcohol on family and social life may not be entirely negative, however. Steinglass[12] has noted the use of alcohol in everyday habits, short-term problem solving and family rituals. While in some families alcohol increases problems in others its use may assist family functioning and play a part in maintaining family stability.

Child abuse

Excessive drinking is also commonly linked to child abuse. An analysis of child abuse cases in the NSPCC (National Society for the Prevention of Cruelty to Children) files found that heavy drinking was a feature in 20 per cent of the families involved.[13] Another study noted an association in metropolitan areas between rates of taking children into care and offences of drunkenness.[14]

*Recommendation No. 4*

It is recommended that social services departments should instruct their social workers to enquire into the drinking behaviour of client families, (especially those where child abuse or family dispute is the presenting problem) so that it is possible to estimate the contribution that alcohol makes to these problems.

▶ Alcohol and employment

Inappropriate alcohol consumption can cause problems for employers, the drinking employee and non drinking colleagues. The employer is harmed by loss of profits and productivity through bad timekeeping, sickness absenteeism, loss of efficiency (alertness, accuracy and judgement), increased risk of accidents, loss of trained staff, bad work discipline and petty crime. The drinking employee stands to suffer loss of pay and promotion, injuries from accidents, physical and mental illness loss of self respect and ultimately loss of job and family. Non drinking colleagues of the employee are exposed to increased accident risk caused by the problem employee and are persistently inconvenienced by the need to rectify or otherwise cover up faults, shoddiness and omissions in the work of the problem drinker.[15] The size of these problems is difficult to quantify.

The timing of workplace accidents is clustered suspiciously around the periods after lunch and the late evening[16] and studies in a Scottish firm showed that 20 per cent of all accidents notified were alcohol-related.[17] The few individuals who were identified as having an alcohol problem had an accident rate some 50 per cent higher than the workplace average.

The 1980 OPCS (Office of Population, Censuses and Surveys) survey of drinking[18] found that 7 per cent of males reported having had a hangover at work in the three months before the survey. Attitudes to alcohol among workers suggest this behaviour will be difficult to change. In another survey,[19] 15 per cent of workers thought it acceptable for someone to come into work regularly with a hangover and almost three-quarters thought it reasonable to drink two pints of beer or half a bottle of wine in a working day lunchtime.

One estimate of the cost to industry of alcohol-related sickness and absenteeism in males was £779 million (1987 prices).[20] This figure would have been far greater if costs of alcohol-related accidents and reduced efficiency at work, which could be £1500 million,[21] had been included.

## ▶ The economic cost of alcohol-related problems

There have been repeated attempts to estimate the economic cost of alcohol to the country, but the exercise is fraught with technical problems. Some of the costs (and benefits) are difficult to define, much of the necessary data is not available, and valuing the social costs is extremely difficult. The calculations of A. Maynard et al.[22] who arrived at a figure of £1990 million for the elements they were able to cost, are shown in Table 3.1. Had they been able to include the uncosted elements, the figure would have been very much greater.

There are economic benefits to be set against these costs. Some, such as tax revenue and employment, are relatively easy to quantify while others, such as the indirect economic and social benefits arising from drinking, are extremely difficult to measure. The population chooses to spend £17 billion on alcoholic

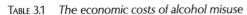

TABLE 3.1    *The economic costs of alcohol misuse*

|  |  | Million £s |
|---|---|---:|
| 1. | Social cost to industry | |
|  | Sickness absence | 779.3 |
|  | Housework services | 52.4 |
|  | Unemployment | 179.6 |
|  | Premature death | 703.7 |
| 2. | *Social cost to National Health Service* | |
|  | Psychiatric in-patient costs | 21.4 |
|  | Non psychiatric in-patient costs | 97.1 |
|  | GP visits | 2.3 |
| 3. | *Responses to alcohol problems* | |
|  | National bodies and research | 1.0 |
| 4. | *Road traffic accidents* | 112.0 |
| 5. | *Social costs of criminal activity* | |
|  | Police involvement in traffic offences | 20.9 |
|  | Drink offences court cases | 19.5 |
|  | *Total costed elements* | |
|  | (including unemployment and premature death) | 1989.1 |
|  | (excluding unemployment and premature death) | 1105.9 |
| 6. | *Uncosted elements* | |
|  | Alcohol-related accidents in home and at work | |
|  | Alcohol-related fire | |
|  | Alcohol-related criminal activity (except drunkenness offences) | |
|  | Reduced productivity at work due to alcohol | |
|  | Costs to social services and other agencies arising from alcohol-related family disputes, child neglect, etc. | |
|  | Emotional pain and suffering from alcohol-related problems. | |

drinks,[23] which suggests that they consider the personal and indirect benefits to themselves are of this magnitude.

*Recommendation No. 5*

It is recommended that econometric studies should be commissioned to ascertain, more comprehensively than has currently been undertaken, the indirect costs and benefits of alcohol use.

## ▶ Strategies for prevention

There are two approaches to the prevention of disease. One is to identify those individuals within a population who are at highest risk and to persuade them to modify that risk. The other is to identify the root cause of a disease incidence in the population and to control that cause. The two approaches are not mutually exclusive, each having complementary advantages and disadvantages which have been widely debated in the field of blood pressure, cholesterol, and cardiovascular disease.[24, 25, 26]

It is ironic that clearly-defined conditions (such as coronary heart disease), which each have a number of interacting risk factors, should inspire attempts at prevention which have a higher profile than those attempts directed against a single (and so more amenable) entity such as alcohol consumption, which plays a significant, if complex, role in the causation of a wide range of illness and mortality.

## ▶ Alcohol consumption as a risk factor

Alcohol consumption, whether considered at an individual level or by population, is linked with a spectrum of harm that has been reviewed in this report and others.[27, 28, 29] The wide variety of alcohol's ill-effects despite attempts to aggregate and describe the overall damage that is done[30, 31, 32, 33, 34, 35] denies them the public concern that is aroused by the effect of diagnostically distinct diseases.

It is now accepted that alcohol consumption displays the characteristics of a risk factor for many of the various forms of harm with which it is associated. In some instances the relationship is less direct and is modified by other influences. Cultural differences in the incidence of social harm, may arise in societies with similar average levels of consumption, as a result of the different behaviours that these societies have learned to associate with alcohol consumption.[36,37,38] In general, however, risk of alcohol-associated harm increases with overall levels of consumption. Levels of alcohol consumption and indicators of alcohol-related harm tend to vary together over time both in England and Wales (see Figure 3.3) and elsewhere.

The small section of the population who are encountering severe difficulties with alcohol are readily identifiable by the remainder of the population. It is human nature to dissociate oneself from such a spectacle, and 'alcoholism' is still popularly viewed as an affliction suffered by a group of the population that is in some way different from the rest. This concept was first seriously challenged in 1956 when Ledermann[39] suggested that distribution of alcohol consumption in a population could be described by a simple mathematical formula. He proposed that alcohol consumption was distributed as shown in Figure 3.4 which shows a log-normal distribution. The quasi-mathematical relationship between population consumption and prevalence of heavy use has been criticised ever since,[40,41] although the existence of some sort of relationship is not in doubt.[42,43,44]

That debate, however, diverts attention from the main issue. It is alcohol consumption that is the risk factor, not alcohol dependence. Alcohol-related harm is proportional to the amount consumed and not to prevalence of 'alcoholism'.[45,46] Even low levels of overall alcohol consumption are associated with increased risk and it has been said that the small number of heavy drinkers are only a minority of those harmed by alcohol.[47] The alcohol problem conforms to the principle that a large number of people at small risk will generate far more ill-health than small numbers at high risk,[48] and it is in these terms that alcohol consumption should be seen as a matter of concern for the public health.

FIGURE 3.3 *The relationship between indicators of harm and alcohol consumption in England and Wales*

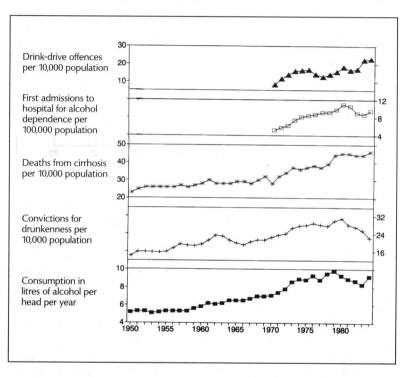

Note that as consumption increases indicators of harm also tend to increase.

Data on consumption and drunkenness and cirrhosis are for the UK, drink–drive offences data is for Britain, and psychiatric admission data for England. The base denominator population used is those aged 15 and over, except for cirrhosis where the total population is used.

SOURCES   Royal College of Psychiatrists, *Alcohol – our favourite drug* (1986); Royal College of Psychiatrists, *Alcohol and alcoholism* (1979).

FIGURE 3.4   *The Ledermann curve*

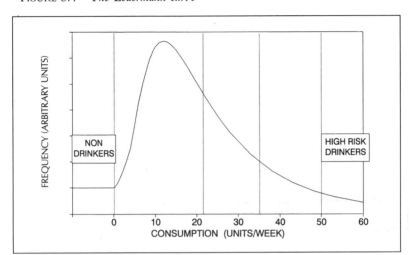

The theoretical (log normal) distribution of levels of consumption in a population. This is very similar to the distributions which are typically observed.

## ▶ High risk versus population strategies

In terms of prevention there are two major strategies: either to target preventive activity on those identified as being heavy drinkers (the high risk approach), or to attempt to reduce consumption across the whole population. Where harm is associated with heavy consumption in certain specific situations it may best be reduced by limiting the amount consumed in those situations; when driving a car, for example, or at football games. Limitation of drinking in these very specific situations may not be reflected in or influenced by levels of overall consumption.

A population strategy of prevention has weighty advantages over the high risk approach. First there is greater potential for a large reduction of harm. One estimate is that an overall reduction to 70 per cent of current intake would have the same effect as if there were a universal observance of currently described safe limits of consumption.[49] This parallels work in other fields which has estimated, for instance, that an overall reduction of blood pressure by 10 per cent would reduce coronary heart disease mortality by 21 per cent, which is similar to the effect that would result from total elimination of high blood pressure (defined as a blood pressure $> 90$ mm Hg in diastole).[50] Secondly, the population approach would aim to change the perception of what levels of drinking are 'normal' (a euphemism for 'common') and such a change would have important corollaries. An environment in which light drinking is the norm would exert a powerful pressure on heavy-drinking individuals to reduce their consumption, and so potentiate the high risk strategy. A change in social drinking habits would demand changes in the alcohol industry to suit these habits, such as the production of increasing ranges of alcohol-free drinks, for example, and altered advertising approaches.

Population strategies do have the disadvantage that they are subject to the 'prevention paradox'. It is unfortunately true that preventive measures which bring much benefit to the population in aggregate offer little to each participating individual,[51] which results in poor motivation to reduce drinking on health grounds. Dr Samuel Johnson recognised the need to stress benefits to the individual in promoting moderation when he wrote, 'To insist against drunkenness as a crime, because it debases reason . . . would be of no service to the common people: but to tell them that they may die in a fit of drunkenness, and shew them how dreadful that would be, cannot fail to make a deep impression'.[52]

The 'high risk' approach to alcohol consumption can complement the population strategy but by itself it is not sufficient. Concentrating attention and services on a few individuals whose drinking patterns place them at very high risk may produce some benefit for these individuals but has the disadvantage of seeming to confirm as acceptable the drinking habits which continue to put most of society at risk. This approach may fit the traditional model of medical care in which the physician, by diagnosis of a problem and prescription of a course of action, turns the person who consults him or her into a patient. For the patient, adoption of a 'sick' role offers some advantages, at the cost of accepting the imposition of a behaviour that both they themselves and their associates consider abnormal. For society, ascribing the sick role to some heavy-drinking individuals has the major drawback of seeming to excuse the majority from the need to consider their own drinking habits.

*Recommendation No. 6*

It is recommended that all those concerned to limit the harm to public health by alcohol should realise that alcohol consumption is a risk factor for alcohol-related harm and should adopt a population strategy to reduce the harm. They should adopt a strategy which aims to shift all members of the population into lower risk levels by reducing consumption.

*Recommendation No. 7*

It is recommended that the population strategy needs to be complemented by a high risk strategy. This strategy seeks to identify individuals within the population who are at extra high risk because of their drinking behaviour and to offer appropriate services to these individuals.

## ▶ The relative importance of alcohol and other drugs

Anyone looking at the relative amounts of government literature and other activity devoted to misuse of alcohol compared to that devoted to misuse of opiates and other addictive drugs might be excused for concluding that alcohol problems were relatively unimportant. It is therefore salutary to try to compare the harm caused by these substances. Addictive drugs other than alcohol and tobacco cause less than 500 deaths per year,[53] that is, one-fiftieth of the probable deaths attributable to alcohol. The contribution of misuse of illegal drugs to hospital admissions and general practice workload are difficult to estimate but are clearly an order of magnitude smaller than that due to alcohol. Similarly, while the effect of illegal drug use on workplace productivity is not negligible it is much smaller than the effect of alcohol and public disorder associated with illegal drug use is far less common than that associated with alcohol use. Tranquilliser related problems affect more people than problems related to use of opiates and other illegal drugs but are still much less common than problems related to alcohol use. One must conclude that the repeated emphasis on problems due to opiates and other illegal drugs owes more to political considerations than to an informed assessment of public health needs.

References

1. B. W. Jeffs and W. M. Saunders 'Minimising alcohol-related offences by enforcing the existing licensing legislation', *British Journal of Addiction*, 78(1983) pp. 67–77.
2. N. Heather, 'Relationships between delinquency and drunkenness among Scottish young offenders', *British Journal of Alcoholism*, 16(1981) pp. 50–61.
3. T. Bennet and R. Wright, 'The relationship between alcohol use and burglary', *British Journal of Addiction*, 79(1984) pp. 431–7.
4. N. Heather, 'Alcohol dependence and problem drinking in Scottish offenders', *British Journal on Alcohol and Alcoholism*, 17(1982) pp. 145–54.
5. H. Gilles, 'Homicide in the West of Scotland', *British Journal of Psychiatry*, 128(1976) pp. 105–27.
6. Home Office (Chairman Baroness Masham), *Report of the working party on young people and alcohol* (London:HMSO, 1987).
7. T. Myers, 'Alcohol and violent crime re-examined: Self reports from two sub-groups of Scottish Male prisoners', *British Journal of Addiction*, 77(1982) pp. 399–413.
8. T. Bennet and R. Wright, op. cit.
9. I. C. Buchan, E. G. Buckley, G. L. S. Deacon, R. Irvine and R. Ryan, 'Problem drinkers and their problems', *Journal of the Royal College of General Practitioners*, 31(1981) pp. 151–3.
10. J. J. Gayford, 'Wife battering a preliminary survey of 100 cases', *British Medical Journal*, 1(1975) pp. 194–7.
11. C. J. Hamilton and J. J. Collins, 'The role of alcohol in wife beating and child abuse: A review of the literature', in J. J. Collins (ed.) *Drinking and Crime* (New York: Guilford Press, 1981).
12. P. Steinglass, *The alcoholic family. Drinking problems in a family context* (London: Hutchinson, 1988).
13. S. J. Creighton, *Trends in child abuse* (London: NSPCC publications, 1984).
14. C. Goodman, *Children in Care*, (Unpublished report to Newcastle City Council, 1986).

15. J. Crofton, 'Extent and costs of alcohol problems in employment: a review of British Data', *Alcohol and alcoholism*, 22(1987) pp. 321–5.
16. M. A. Argyropoulos-Grisanos and P. J. L. Hawkins, *Alcohol and Industrial Accidents* (London: Christian Economic and Social Research Foundation, 1980).
17. P. B. Beaumont and S. J. Allsop, 'The Beverage Report', *Occupational Safety and Health*, 13(1983) pp. 25–7.
18. P. Wilson, *Drinking in England and Wales* (London: OPCS Social Survey Division, HMSO, 1980).
19. R. Roberts, R. Cyster and J. McEwen, 'Alcohol Consumption and the Workplace: Prospects for change', *Public Health*, 102(1988) pp. 463–9.
20. D. Robinson, A. Maynard and R. Chester, *Controlling Legal Addictions* (London: Macmillan, 1989).
21. E. G. Lucas, 'Alcohol in industry', *British Medical Journal*, 294(1987) pp. 460–1.
22. D. Robinson, A. Maynard and R. Chester, op. cit.
23. Central Statistical Office, *Annual abstract of statistics*, No. 125 (London: HMSO, 1989).
24. J. Shepherd, D. J. Betteridge, P. Durrington, M. Laker, B. Lewis, J. Mann, J. P. D. Reckless and G. R. Thompson, 'Strategies for reducing coronary heart disease and desirable limits for blood lipid concentrations: guidelines of the British Hyperlipdaemia Association', *British Medical Journal*, 295(1987) pp. 1245–6.
25. B. Lewis, J. Mann and M. Mancini, 'Reducing the risks of coronary heart disease in individuals and in the population', *Lancet*, i(1986) pp. 956–9.
26. W. B. Kannel, J. D. Neaton, D. Wentworth, H. E. Thomas, J. Stanber, S. B. Hulley and M. O. Kjelsberg, 'Overall and coronary heart disease mortality rates in relation to major risk factors in 325,342 men screened for the MRFIT', *American Heart Journal*, 112(1986) pp. 825–36.
27. Royal College of Physicians, *A great and growing evil. The medical consequences of alcohol abuse* (London: Tavistock, 1987).
28. Royal College of General Practitioners, *Alcohol – a balanced view*. Reports from general practice 24 (London: Royal College of General Practitioners, 1986).
29. Royal College of Psychiatrists, *Alcohol – our favourite drug* (London: Tavistock, 1986).
30. *A great and growing evil*, op. cit
31. *Alcohol – a balanced view*, op. cit.
32. *Alcohol – our favourite drug*, op. cit.
33. P. Anderson, 'Excess mortality associated with alcohol consumption', *British Medical Journal*, 297(1988) pp. 824–6.

34. R. McDonnell and A. Maynard, 'Estimation of the life years lost from alcohol-related premature death', *Alcohol and alcoholism*, 20(1985) pp. 435–43.
35. Office of Health Economics, *Alcohol – Reducing the harm*. Studies of current health problems No. 70 (London: Office of Health Economics, 1981).
36. *A great and growing evil*, op. cit.
37. *Alcohol – our favourite drug*, op. cit.
38. World Health Organisation, *Problems related to alcohol consumption* (Geneva: WHO Technical report series, no. 650, 1980).
39. S. Ledermann, 'Alcool, Alcoolisme, Alcoolisation. Données Scientifiques de Caractère Physiologique Economique et Social', *Institut National d'Etudes Démographiques Travaux et Documents*. Cahier No. 29 (Paris: Presses Universitaires de France, 1956).
40. H. Mulford and J. Fitzgerald, 'Per capita alcohol sales, heavy drinkers prevalence, and alcohol problems in Iowa for 1958–1985', *British Journal of Addictions*, 83(1988) pp. 265–8.
41. J. Duffy and S. Cohen, 'Total alcohol consumption and excessive drinking', *British Journal of Addictions*, 73(1978) pp. 259–64.
42. WHO, *Problems related to alcohol consumption*, op. cit.
43. R. E. Kendell, 'Alcoholism: a medical or a political problem?', *British Medical Journal*, i(1979) pp. 367–71.
44. M. Hilton, 'Trends in drinking problems and attitudes in the United States: 1979–1984', *British Journal of Addictions*, 83(1988) pp. 1421–7.
45. K. Bruun et al., *Alcohol control policies in public health perspective* (Helsinki: Finnish Foundation for Alcohol studies, 1975).
46. L. de Lint and W. Schmidt, 'Consumption averages and alcoholism prevalence. A brief review of Epidemiological investigations', *British Journal of Addictions*, 66(1971) pp. 97–107.
47. N. Kreitman, 'Alcohol consumption and the preventive paradox', *British Journal of Addictions*, 81(1986) pp. 353–63.
48. G. Rose, 'Sick Individuals and Sick Populations', *International Journal of Epidemiology*, 14(1985) pp. 32–8.
49. N. Kreitman, *Alcohol consumption and the preventative paradox*, op. cit.
50. G. Rose, 'Sick Individuals and Sick Populations', op. cit.
51. G. Rose, 'Strategy of prevention: lessons from cardiovascular disease', *British Medical Journal*, 282(1981) pp. 1847–51.
52. Dr Samuel Johnson, (1763). Quoted in Boswell, *Life of Johnson* (Unabridged) (Oxford University Press, 1980) p. 325.
53. A. Maynard, G. Hardman and A. Whelan, 'Measuring the costs of addictive substances', *British Journal of Addiction*, 82(1987) pp. 701–6.

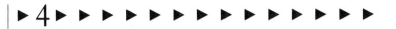

# ▶4▶ ▶ ▶ ▶ ▶ ▶ ▶ ▶ ▶ ▶ ▶ ▶

# A BETTER-INFORMED PUBLIC

▶ How much can I drink without damaging my health?

A generally agreed guideline for safe drinking is:

*Weekly intake*

| | MEN | WOMEN |
|---|---|---|
| Low risk | Less than 21 units | Less than 14 units |
| Increasing risk | 22–50 units | 15–35 units |
| High risk | Above 50 units | Above 35 units |

A unit of drink consists of half a pint of ordinary strength beer, or a glass of wine, or a single measure of spirits; each of which contains about 8 gm of alcohol – for a fuller definition see Introduction, page 2. These figures have been agreed by all bodies active in the field[1,2,3] and this is a great improvement on the previous situation, where different authorities quoted different guidelines.

Some people question the use of guidelines[4] on the grounds that they are entirely arbitrary and may encourage those currently drinking at levels below those of the guideline to drink more. Also, the arbitrary nature of guidelines cannot be disputed. There is a continuum of risk running from no risk of harm at no alcohol intake to very high risk of harm at high alcohol intake. People with low alcohol intakes still have a slightly increased risk and there is no cut-off point below which there is no risk (see Chapter 3).

## ► Individual variation

Guidelines may also be criticised for taking no account of individual variation apart from gender. The rise in blood alcohol level after drinking a unit of drink is affected by the rate at which alcohol is absorbed, the size of the body water pool (large in large individuals), the rate at which alcohol is excreted by the kidneys, and the rate at which it is metabolised in the body. All these things vary considerably between individuals. Sensitivity to the toxic effects of alcohol varies and, for example, people with certain genetic markers on their blood white cells (B8 or DR3 HLA antigens) are more susceptible to liver damage by alcohol than people without.[5] Individuals also vary in the way their central nervous systems respond to raised blood alcohol levels. Tolerance, whereby co-ordination is less severely impaired by high blood alcohol levels in heavy drinkers than in less experienced drinkers, is a well-recognised phenomenon.

These objections to general guidelines are valid but the question, 'How much can I drink without harming my health?' is still a natural one and it does not help if an answer is not forthcoming. Safer drinking guidelines represent a sensible compromise and help people to judge the healthiness of their own drinking behaviour. If everyone regulated their drinking by these guidelines there is no doubt that the damage to public health due to alcohol would be dramatically reduced.

## ► Informed choice

Informed choice is a prerequisite for sensible drinking, as it is for all other aspects of healthy living. What information does an individual need to have in order to make an informed choice about personal drinking habits? Members of the public need to know the effect that alcohol has on their bodies. The safer drinking guidelines discussed earlier in this chapter are clearly one part of this information, but people also need to know how their short-term physical and social skills and their long-term health can be affected by alcohol.

Individuals also need to know the approximate alcohol content of the drinks that they consume so that they can monitor their own intake. This has become more difficult as the diversity of alcoholic drinks available has increased. For example, the alcohol content of different beers varies from 3 per cent to 8 per cent. Estimating volume may also be difficult as non-standard pack sizes become increasingly common. Ways in which better labelling can allow people to make informed choices will be discussed in Chapter 10. There are also a large number of myths about alcohol that people need to recognise as false. Informed choice only becomes a reality when people have adequate knowledge. Only then can they estimate the consequences of their alcohol intake and decide for themselves drinking patterns which will increase their enjoyment of life rather than make it a misery.

Some health educators have wanted to present alcohol as a substance whose only effects are harmful and objected to any admission that some effects of alcohol use are beneficial.[6] The temptation to propagandise must be avoided since it violates the principle of informed choice and lacks credibility. The harm resulting from use of alcohol is real enough and far too frequent, so there is no need to overstate the case.

## ▶ Personal responsibility versus society's responsibility

The corollary of informed choice is personal responsibility. There is no escape from the need for everyone to look after their own health and avoid drinking patterns which they know will cause damage. Society cannot, however, unload all responsibility for public health on to its members. Informed choice requires not only that the individual should be informed, but that such choice should be available, and the individual should be able to make that choice free from undue cultural and environmental pressures.

The tension between personal responsibility and the responsibility of society towards its members is reflected in health promotion strategies (see Table 4.1).[7] Traditional health education has laid emphasis on the individual's responsibility and sought to change behaviour through change in knowledge, skills and attitudes. The theoretical, practical and ideological limitations of this approach to health promotion have been forcibly

TABLE 4.1    *Models of health education*

| MODEL | BEHAVIOURAL CHANGE | SELF EMPOWERMENT | COLLECTIVE ACTION |
|---|---|---|---|
| Aim | To improve health by changing individual behaviour. | To improve health by developing people's ability to understand and control their health status as far as possible within the constraints of their environment. | To improve health by changing environmental, social and economic factors by community involvement and action. |
| Model of Health | Optimum biological functioning and role performance. | Spiritual, physical, mental and social harmony. Individual feeling of active well-being. Adaptation, happiness, high self-esteem and positive self-concept. | Health is a socially-defined concept related to group norms. Outcome of interplay between environmental, social and economic influences. |
| Model of Education | Classical humanist education is an assimilative process of pre-defined knowledge, values and standards. | Progressivist education is about experiment and discovery. Education should encourage questioning. | Reconstructionist education is the main agent of social change pursued through projects and problem-solving. |
| Examples of Methods | Propaganda. Mass media. Attitude modification. Self management. Administrative and legislative change. | Lifeskills training. Value clarification. Self-help groups (coping). Counselling. Pastoral care. | Advocacy. Consciousness. Self-help groups (campaigning). Pressure groups. Administrative and legislative change. |

| MODEL | BEHAVIOURAL CHANGE | SELF EMPOWERMENT | COLLECTIVE ACTION |
|---|---|---|---|
| Use in Alcohol Field | Posters and leaflets. Knowledge of alcohol content of drinks and of the effects of alcohol on body. Requiring better labelling of alcoholic drinks. | Drinkwatchers. AA groups. Relaxation groups. Assertiveness training. | Campaigns for enforcement of licensing laws and for cheaper alcohol-free drinks and non-drinking leisure facilities. CADD (Campaign Against Drinking and Driving). |

SOURCE  Modified from J. French and L. Adams, 'From analysis to synthesis – Theories of Health Education', *Health Education Journal*, 45(1986).

criticised.[8] Community action instead concentrates on the physical, social and cultural environment in which the individual lives and seeks to modify that environment in such a way as to improve the individual's health. In the context of reducing harm to health through alcohol they would seek to reduce the pressures which lead an individual to drink in a health-damaging fashion and to increase the opportunities to obtain enjoyment and fulfilment without heavy consumption of alcohol. Though frequently presented as alternative strategies, the individual behavioural change approach and the community action approach should be seen as complementary to each other. This report advocates a combination of both approaches.

## ▶ Attitudes to drinking

Drinking behaviour is influenced by a complex set of attitudes and much risky behaviour can be traced back to unhealthy attitudes. Examples of such unhelpful attitudes are shown in Figure 4.1. The frequent association in Western culture between hospitality, friendliness, generosity and the offering and consumption of alcohol can make it extremely difficult for an individual to regulate alcohol intake. Normative views on alcohol consumption and attitudes that those who decline offers

FIGURE 4.1

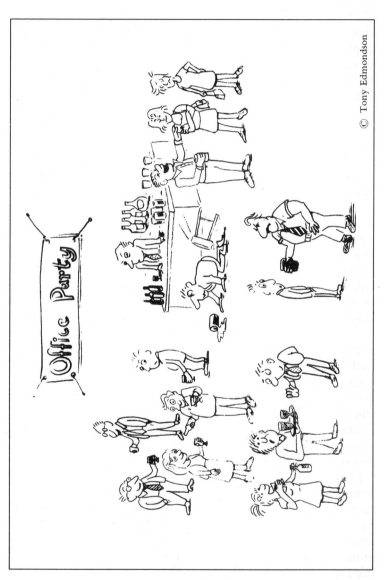

of drink are peculiar, abnormal or unmanly can also exert great pressures on an individual to drink more than they would otherwise wish. These attitudes have become embedded in the culture so that they are often not noticed. The host may not think to provide non-alcoholic alternatives, and drinks are bought in rounds so that one's consumption is determined by the size of the group and not by one's own wishes. Intoxication may become a way of identifying with one's peer group and gaining favourable attention.

Unhealthy attitudes to one's own drinking may be coupled with unhealthy attitudes to those whom everyone (except maybe themselves) recognises as having a drink problem. It is not helpful to view 'alcoholics' as a breed apart, whose misfortunes are irrelevant to the drinking patterns of everyone else and who are totally different from 'social drinkers'. Attitudes of this sort are often held with great tenacity despite the repeated everyday experience which shows that most of the unfavourable consequences of alcohol consumption are experienced by those who are not 'alcoholics' (see Chapter 3).

Inappropriate beliefs about those who have severe problems with drink are important and damaging to public health for three reasons: first, because they make it difficult for individuals to make healthy choices about their own drinking behaviour; second, because they make it more difficult for those with problems to reintegrate themselves into the community; and third, because they make it more difficult to obtain political support for effective programmes to reduce the harmful consequences of alcohol consumption. Health education, coupled with other health promotion activities, must aim first to increase knowledge about alcohol and drinking and second to change unhealthy attitudes to drinking and to people with alcohol-related problems.

The health education task will be long and difficult. Unhealthy attitudes and false mythology about alcohol are deeply entrenched. Health promotion in relation to smoking offers an encouraging precedent. It has taken thirty years to change attitudes and behaviour but now smokers are in a minority and attitudes are becoming increasingly unfavourable to smoking. The issues related to alcohol are more complicated but even here there are signs of movement such as the undoubted change in attitudes to drinking and driving.

*Recommendation No. 8*

It is recommended that a comprehensive health education programme on alcohol should be instituted. This programme should cover guidelines for safe drinking, knowledge of the effects of alcohol on the body, understanding of the social and cultural contexts in which alcohol is used and social skills so that people are able to resist pressures to drink when they would rather not do so.

*Recommendation No. 9*

It is recommended that alcohol education should not concentrate exclusively on the individual's responsibility for his or her own behaviour but should also encourage people to examine their own cultural and physical environment in order to identify those factors which pressure individuals into consuming alcohol and those factors which support decisions to drink responsibly.

Health education activities may focus on alcohol alone or consider alcohol as one item in a whole lifestyle approach. They may be short-term (days or weeks) or a long-term (years) programmes of activity. They may be planned or opportunistic, formal or informal, and 'expert'-lead or client-lead.

## ▶ Evaluation of alcohol education and health promotion

Before discussing examples of these approaches we need to decide what their objectives were and how they should be evaluated.

Behavioural objectives might be to reduce the overall consumption of alcohol, to reduce the numbers of people driving after drinking, or to increase the number of people with alcohol-related problems who seek help for those problems. Often such behavioural objectives are unrealistic and objectives need to be set in terms of changing attitude, increasing knowledge or merely raising awareness. Measures of activities under-taken (process) such as numbers of people attending events, numbers of people requesting further information, and reactions of members of the target audience or staff are also helpful in evaluating these activities.

As with other health promotions, it is difficult to decide whether any observed change in knowledge, attitudes or behaviour is the result of an alcohol education activity. Causal inferences can be made with most confidence if a formal experimental design with a control group has been used, as was the case in the HEA (Health Education Authority) schools project[9] but usually this is not practical. Studies of the association of changes in knowledge, attitudes and behaviour with exposure to and awareness of alcohol education activities may also suggest whether the health promotion activity has contributed to any changes observed.

Formal evaluation of alcohol education has usually given disappointing results.[10] However, alcohol education is usually attempting to influence attitudes which have been ingrained over many years and it is unreasonable to expect a day, a week or even a year of activity to totally reverse these attitudes. Alcohol education activities should not be rejected because they do not immediately prevent all alcohol-related harm.

## ▶ Drinkwise Day – a single-focus event

Drinkwise events aim to promote sensible attitudes to drinking, to make facts about alcohol and its effects widely known and to advise on safe limits and how to keep within them. One such Drinkwise event was held in London for a week in 1986.[11] Local radio and television stations devoted several programmes to alcohol, posters were displayed in the London Underground, stalls were set up where members of the public could test their knowledge of alcohol with a quiz and collect literature on alcohol, and professional groups such as social workers, nurses, doctors and managers attended conferences on alcohol and its public health implications. Similar events have been held else-where and Drinkwise Day has now become an annual national event, the first being held in 1989. The organisation of a Drinkwise event will be discussed in Chapter 9.

Short-term events are unpopular with some health educators, who rightly point out that attitude and habit change are complex processes which are more likely to be influenced by sustained activity. There is probably little point in mounting single-focus events if no attempt is made to follow them up. On the other hand, short-term events can be very effective in generating interest and raising the profile of an alcohol education programme and sowing seeds which can be nurtured by follow-up activities. They also have the great advantage that many people can be persuaded to make a short-term commitment who would not contribute to a sustained lower profile activity. The advantage *and* disadvantage of short-term events is that people can see that 'something is being done'. This is an advantage because it is very good for building the morale of those interested in prevention of alcohol-related harm, but it is also a disadvantage because it may satisfy those who only want a token response and divert energies from a sustained lower-profile programme.

## ▶ Tyne Tees alcohol education campaign

The aims of this campaign were to promote sensible drinking and help people to recognise their drinking problems and seek help. It was run in the North East from 1974–84 and managed by a committee of District Medical Officers, Health Education Officers and representatives of the North East Council on Alcoholism, the Regional Addiction Treatment Unit and the Health Education Council. The campaign strategy included education and training for field workers, and education for the general public through radio, television, press, exhibitions, talks and workshops.[12]

The campaign was generally judged to be successful but the evaluation[13] identified features which would need extra attention in future activities. The high-profile activities generated considerable community interest, to which front line health educators such as school teachers, health education officers, specialist alcohol workers, health visitors, and so on, had to respond. A training programme with a manual and key tutors was set up to help them fulfil this role but even more preparation would have been helpful.

The campaign also generated a large demand for services, with many new clients seeking help from the specialist alcohol agencies. This was one of the objectives of the campaign but the size of the response was larger than anticipated and the agencies found it difficult to respond adequately.

## ▶ Alcohol education as part of personal and social education (PSE)

Alcohol education ought to be included in general education. One response to this need has been to invite an outside speaker (possibly a doctor or a member of Alcoholics Anonymous) into a school to deliver a lecture on the terrible consequences of drinking too much alcohol. Not surprisingly, this approach has achieved little. Such isolated interventions were unrelated to all other school activities, often in conflict with a child's own experience at home, and made no concession to the child's autonomy.

Much more successful and educationally sound is the inclusion of alcohol issues in the broad topic of personal and social education (PSE). Choices about alcohol are seen as one of the many choices that an individual has to make along with choices about sexual behaviour, drug use, smoking, eating, exercise and other health-related behaviour. The aim is to equip the child with the information and skills that will enable it to retain maximum control over its own life and grow into a complete healthy adult.[14] This approach infiltrates not only special lessons but all parts of the curriculum and the extracurricular activity of the school.

Integration of alcohol education into school activity is likely to be more effective but it will be many years before the benefits are apparent. Some people are uneasy with the PSE approach because it may appear value-free. However, alcohol issues are usually considered in the value framework of seeking to fulfil one's own mental, physical and social potential and of showing consideration for others. It may also be noted that the PSE approach is very similar to that used by behavioural skills-trained alcohol counsellors to help clients with alcohol-related problems.[15]

The new national curriculum for schools in the United Kingdom[16] requires that health education issues, including alcohol, must be covered as part of the core subjects. This development is to be welcomed both because it gives government recognition to the importance of the subject and because the subject should now be covered in those schools which have previously neglected it.

## ▶ Alcohol issues in the Look After Your Heart! (LAYH!) campaign

The LAYH! campaign is an example of a multi-issue community campaign and despite its name is concerned with promotion of healthy lifestyles rather than the narrow aim of disease prevention. Drinking is covered, along with eating, smoking, stress, exercise and checking for risk factors. Presenting alcohol issues in this way may be more effective since they are seen in the context of health and fitness rather than as an isolated issue which many people may find threatening.

Community participation could be a prominent feature of the LAYH!, though this approach has not been fully developed. In other cardiovascular prevention campaigns such as the North Karelia project[17] and the Stanford project[18] a commitment to real community involvement and participation seems to have greatly increased the effectiveness of the health promotion.

## ▶ Media alcohol campaigns

Drink-driving campaigns with short advertisements on television and posters on hoardings are a regular feature before Christmas in the United Kingdom and campaigns on other alcohol issues are occasionally mounted (Figure 4.2). This sort of campaign is very expensive and many health educators doubt whether it is effective. On the other hand, media campaigns may be attractive to government departments because they are very visible and enable the department to say that they are taking action to reduce the problem.

The evidence suggests that mass media campaigns will usually not change behaviours[19, 20, 21] but if carefully focused, sustained and integrated with other health-promotion activities they may facilitate changes in attitudes to alcohol and problem drinking.

## ▶ Informal discussion as part of routine medical contact

Doctors and medical staff in general practice and in hospitals should be alert to the possibility that their patients may be drinking in a high risk fashion and should be prepared to discuss the subject in a non-judgmental fashion. There are suggestions that this type of opportunistic informal health education is highly effective.[22] It will be discussed further in Chapter 8.

---

*Recommendation No. 10*

It is recommended that at a local level health promoters should use a range of methods to promote sensible drinking including short-term 'events' such as Drinkwise Days and sustained low-key, long-term programmes. Alcohol issues can be covered either as an isolated issue or as one component of a healthy lifestyle package.

---

*Recommendation No. 11*

It is recommended that alcohol education programmes should be evaluated in terms of awareness of issues, knowledge retained and attitudes to alcohol and alcohol-related problems, and possibly in terms of drinking behaviour. In evaluating these programmes it is important not to set unrealistic objectives.

---

## ▶ Alcohol in the media

The subject of advertising alcohol in the media will be discussed in Chapter 11. This section deals with the coverage of alcohol

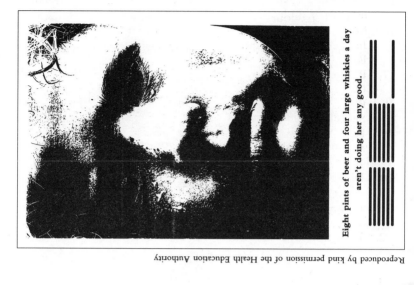

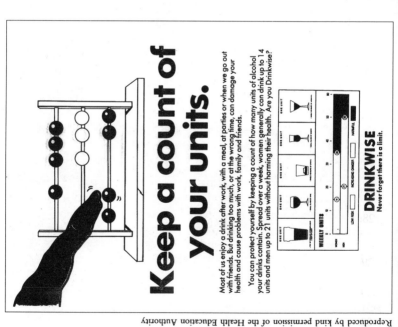

# Keep a count of your units.

Most of us enjoy a drink after work, with a meal, at parties or when we go out with friends. But drinking too much, or at the wrong time, can damage your health and cause problems with work, family and friends.

You can protect yourself by keeping a count of how many units of alcohol your drinks contain. Spread over a week, women generally can drink up to 14 units and men up to 21 units without harming their health. Are you Drinkwise?

**DRINKWISE**
Never forget there is a limit.

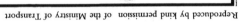

FIGURE 4.2

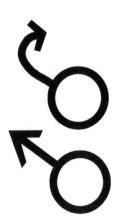

73

and drinking in the general content of press and broadcasting. Drinking behaviour and the norms and values associated with alcohol are socially defined and as such will be influenced not only by parents, peers, schools and everyday experience but also by papers, magazines, radio and television.

An analysis of prime time television (BBC1, BBC2, ITV and Channel 4) showed that alcohol featured in nearly 90 per cent of fictional programmes (see Figure 4.3) but the adverse consequences of alcohol were rarely shown.[23] In non-fictional programmes alcohol was most often portrayed on news features. In these it was usually portrayed in association with a celebration, while in accident and crime reporting the alcohol connection was rarely mentioned.

FIGURE 4.3   *The portrayal of alcohol on prime-time television*

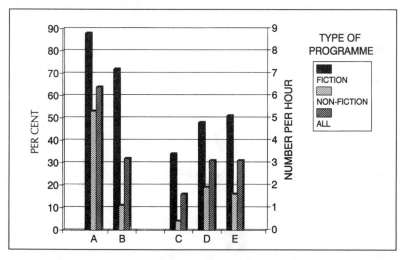

The mentions of alcohol on television programmes between 6.00 and 10.30 pm, April to June 1983 was analysed.

A = Percentage of programmes including reference to alcohol
B = Percentage of programmes showing consumption of alcohol
C = Number of drinking scenes per hour
D = Number of visual references to alcohol per hour
E = Number of verbal references to alcohol per hour

SOURCE A. Hansen, 'The portrayal of alcoholism on television', *Health Education Journal*, 45(1986) pp. 127–31.

No one is suggesting that characters in television soap operas should deliver lectures on the evils of drink every night but there is anxiety that thoughtless portrayal of drinking in storylines may reinforce unhealthy stereotypes. Action in our most popular 'soaps' is centred on public houses and most discussion takes place in situations where alcohol is consumed.

*Recommendation No. 12*

It is recommended that the BBC and the IBA should review their policies to ensure that unhealthy attitudes to drinking and unhelpful stereotypes of problem drinkers are not reinforced by fictional or non-fictional programmes. Viewers should complain when programme contents undermine healthy attitudes to drinking.

## ▶ The need for proper funding for alcohol education

'The trouble with health promotion is not that it has been tried and found wanting but that it has been tried and found to be difficult'. This chapter has warned against unrealistic expectations of health promotion activity and shown that the results of previous health promotion activities related to alcohol have often been disappointing. This should be an argument for redoubling our efforts, not for giving up.

It is most unlikely that health education measures on their own will be sufficient to combat harm to the public health due to alcohol but they certainly have an important contribution to make. However, it is curious that governments which have usually been the most optimistic about the effectiveness of alcohol education have also been reluctant to allocate the resources necessary for such programmes.

So far the resources put into health education generally and alcohol education in particular have been pitiably small. The total budget in 1989 of the Health Education Authority for alcohol and drug education was £644,000 to which very small sums from the district health authorities and the local authorities may be added. These sums have to be set against the £200 million[24] spent by the industry in promoting consumption of alcoholic drinks. The time for allocating a reasonable budget for health education on drinking and alcohol is long overdue.

First, the health education techniques which we already have should be applied much more intensively to prevention of alcohol-related problems, which will require reasonable budgets for staff and materials. Second, we need more effective health education techniques which can only be developed by proper evaluation of new and existing activities. This evaluation will require budgets and staff. If resources were made available, programmes could be developed rapidly by expanding existing alcohol education activities by workers in the Health Education Authority, the district health authorities, the local education authorities and the non statutory agencies.

> ## Recommendation No. 13
>
> It is recommended that the Government should make available earmarked funds for health education related to alcohol. There should be at least one person per health district (approximately 200,000 population) charged with the task of alcohol education. This person may be employed by the health authority or by a voluntary agency contracted to provide this service to the district.

References

1. Health Education Council, *That's the limit* (London: HEC, 1985).
2. Royal College of Psychiatrists, *Alcohol – our favourite drug* (London: Tavistock, 1986).
3. Royal College of Physicians, *A great and growing evil; The medical consequences of alcohol abuse* (London:Tavistock, 1987).
4. R. E. Kendell 'Drinking Sensibly', *British Journal of Addiction*, 82(1987) pp. 1279–88.
5. J. B. Saunders, A. D. Wodak and R. Williams, 'What determines susceptibility to liver damage from alcohol', *Journal of Royal Society of Medicine*, 77(1984) pp. 204–16.
6. R. Roberts, 'Hiccups in alcohol education', *Health Education Journal*, 47(1988) pp. 73–6.

7.  J. French and L. Adams, 'From analysis to synthesis – Theories of Health education', *Health Education Journal*, 45(1986) pp. 71–4.

8.  B. K. Tones, 'Health education: prevention or perversion', *Journal of Royal Society of Health*, 3(1981) pp. 114–17.

9.  G. Bagnall, 'Alcohol education and its evaluation – some key issues', *Health Education Journal*, 46(1987) pp. 162–5.

10. B. N. Kinder, N. E. Pape and S. Walfish, 'Drug and alcohol education programmes: a review of outcome studies', *International Journal of Addictions*, 15(1987) pp. 1035–54.

11. R. Bunton and R. Cyster, 'Drinking wisely in London', *Health Education Journal*, 47(1988) pp. 76–9.

12. I. Simnett, 'A personal perspective on the Tyne Tees Alcohol Education Campaign', *Journal of the Institute of Health Education*, 21(1983) pp. 63–6.

13. J. Budd, P. Gray and R. McCron, *The Tyne Tees Alcohol Education Campaign – An evaluation*, (Leicester University: Centre for Mass Communication Research, 1982).

14. B. K. Tones, 'Health Education, PSE and the question of voluntarism', *Journal of the Institute of Health Education*, 25(1987) pp. 41–52.

15. P. Williamson and H. Norris, *Personal Skills for Problem Drinkers: A Counsellor's Guide*, (Birmingham: Aquarius, 1984).

16. Department of Education and Science, *Science in the National Curriculum*, (London: HMSO, 1989).

17. P. Puska *et al.*, 'The North Karelia youth project: Evaluation of two years of intervention on health behaviour and CVD risk factors among 13–15 year old children', *Preventive Medicine*, 11(1982) pp. 550–70.

18. A. J. Meyer *et al.*, 'Skills training in a cardiovascular health education campaign', *Journal of Consulting and Clinical Psychology*, 48(1980) pp. 129–42.

19. I. Rootman, 'Using health promotion to reduce alcohol problems', in M. Grant (ed.) *Alcohol policies*, European series No. 18 (Copenhagen: WHO Regional Office for Europe, 1985).

20. M. Plant, F. Pirie and N. Kreitman, 'Evaluation of the Scottish Health Education Units 1976 Campaign on alcoholism', *Social Psychiatry*, 14(1979) pp. 11–24.

21. H. T. Blane and L. E. Hewitt, 'Alcohol, public education and mass media: An overview', *Alcohol Health and Research World*, 5(1980) pp. 2–16.

22. P. Wallace, S. Cutler and A. Haines, 'Randomised control trial of General Practitioner intervention in patients with excessive alcohol consumption', *British Medical Journal*, 297(1988) pp. 663–8.

23. A. Hansen, 'The portrayal of alcohol on television', *Health Education Journal*, 45(1986) pp. 127–31.
24. Lancet, 'Dying for a Drink', *Lancet*, ii(1987) pp. 1249–50.

# CONTROL OF AVAILABILITY: LICENSING LAWS

▶ The efficacy of licensing laws

Licensing laws are one strategy by which the state can influence alcohol consumption by its citizens and thereby influence alcohol-related harm. Licensing laws are designed to limit or control the availability of alcohol to the public. They may do this by regulating the minimum age at which alcohol may be purchased, the types of alcohol which can be sold (for example, the recently repealed ban on high-alcohol lager in Iceland), the measures in which it can be sold (for example, prevention of sale of 'liquor by the drink' in some American States), or the times and places at which it can be purchased (the number of alcohol retail outlets available to a population, or the times at which such outlets might be open).

There is much debate about the influence that such laws have on the level of consumption and level of alcohol-related harm in a population. Two national committees which sat in the early 1970s recommended the relaxation of licensing law, as part of a package of measures designed to make the drinking of alcohol a more socially integrated habit.[1,2] In 1978 the DHSS (Department of Health and Social Security) Advisory Committee on Alcoholism concluded that licensing relaxations would have indeterminate consequences.[3] In 1980 the WHO concluded that there was evidence that control over distribution was effective in controlling alcohol consumption and harm.[4]

Many of the uncertainties regarding the efficacy of licensing restrictions are due to the difficulties of isolating their effect from the influence of trends in social attitude and price. Furthermore, it is essential that any discussion of the effect of licensing laws takes into consideration the extent to which they are enforced.

## ▶ Enforcement

The policies by which such laws are enforced govern the impact they have upon society's drinking habits. A law of draconian restriction will have little effect upon alcohol consumption unless it is commonly perceived that transgression will promptly be detected and punishment appropriately administered.

This point was illustrated by a study reported in 1983.[5] In one summer, in agreement with all local licensees, the police of a tourist town adopted a policy of regular visits to licensed premises, to ensure that the laws governing sobriety were being observed. That summer, there was a 20 per cent reduction in arrests, most particularly for those crimes which the study showed to be alcohol-related. The belief that the new policy had produced a real fall in offending was confirmed by a similar decrease in numbers of offences reported to the police by members of the public, and by the absence of such a decrease in a neighbouring town where the policy was not adopted.

The authors of this study reviewed the wide regional variations in policing habits relating to alcohol, and demonstrated the failure of police to enforce some licensing laws. They noted that in Scotland during 1978 there were 12,600 arrests for drunkenness, but very few prosecutions of licensees for selling alcohol to intoxicated customers.

## ▶ Restriction on number of retail outlets

Policies of prohibition will never eliminate all drinking of alcohol, as is shown by the experience of the United States in the prohibition years, and by the current experience of some Islamic countries today. Restriction of access to legal alcohol does, however, reduce consumption to a certain extent, even though it cannot abolish it. During the Polish economic crisis of the early 1980s, alcohol rationing was introduced in 1981 and a sharp reduction in consumption of alcohol was observed despite a fall in the price of alcohol relative to other goods. This reduced consumption was associated with a reduction in admissions to hospital for alcohol-related disorders, and a reduction in admissions to 'sobering up stations'. At the same time, however, there was an increase in sales of non-beverage alcohol (such as methanol) and in cases of toxic poisoning, attributed to the consumption of such fluids.[6]

It has been argued that a change in the number of alcohol retail outlets will only affect consumption in places where such outlets are few relative to the population.[7] The effect of a change in the number of outlets from a low initial concentration was demonstrated in Finland, where a dramatic increase in premises (22 per cent more shops selling alcohol, 32 per cent more restaurants fully licensed, 3000 more cafés selling beer), as well as a reduction in age limit, led to consumption suddenly increasing by 47 per cent.[8] The effect of restrictions to be expected in a country where alcohol retail outlets are already common has been calculated as a decrease of 2 per cent in alcohol consumed for a 1 per cent decrease in the number of licensed premises.[9]

Some have argued against any effect of limiting retail outlets on overall consumption or alcohol-related harm. In 1975, for example, R. E. Popham, W. Schmidt and L. de Lint[10] cited three observations to support this view. First, they found no relationship between indicators of harm and the concentration per population of premises licensed for on-site consumption. Second, there was no difference in indicators of harm between American states operating a licence system and states conducting a monopoly system. However, in reaching these conclusions they made no allowance for other types of retail outlet, for differences in socio-economic structure and in demography, or for policing policy. Third, they reported that no change occurred in indicators of harm after 'diversification' of taverns in Ontario, Canada. However, the changes discussed affected only licences for premises for on-site drinking which catered to relatively wealthy sections of the population. The authors said that control measures (licensing laws) are less influential than policies of taxation. But this sensible observation should not lead to a reliance solely on fiscal measures.

A more modern change in laws of alcohol availability was the reintroduction in parts of one American state of sales of drinks by the glass in restaurants where previously customers wishing to drink with a meal had to bring their own unopened bottle purchased elsewhere (a practice know as 'brown bagging'). This increase in permitted outlets was associated with a rise in overall consumption of distilled spirits[11] and, as a separate analysis showed,[12] an associated increase in alcohol-related accidents.

## ▶ Other restrictions on alcohol sales

The effects of licensing restrictions during the First World War have been studied.[13] In a response to concern about drinking in dockyards and munitions factories, laws were introduced in 1915 to limit opening times of retail and licensed premises, purchase by credit, the alcohol content of spirits, and the 'long pull' – a generous measure of ale. Some parts of the country were affected by these restrictions before others, and in these areas an important short-term effect was shown of reduced public drunkenness and liver cirrhosis mortality. The effect was not universal and was slight in rural areas.

Other factors introduced at this time are likely to have contributed to the observed reduction in alcohol-related problems. These factors were price rises resulting from a limitation of spirit and beer production, and of wine importation, in 1916–1918. The effects of public exhortations against drinking, the example of King George V who gave up alcohol altogether, and the impact of widespread militarisation, could not be adequately accounted for. It is highly probable that changing public opinion nationally, and broadly implemented price rises, swamped any longer-term effect of the licensing laws. Nevertheless, the authors noted that some of the restrictions were retained after the war and neither public drunkenness nor cirrhosis mortality returned to pre-1914 levels.

The effects of changing availability of alcohol have been studied under different circumstances in Sweden where, in 1955, alcohol ceased to be rationed but was made more expensive.[14] The figures for per capita consumption showed a subsequent increase of 50 per cent and mortality from liver cirrhosis quadrupled. The rise in cirrhosis could be explained by a disproportionate increase in the number of heavy drinkers. This shift in distribution of drinking patterns arose because the new increased price of alcohol was more than the previous price for legally-supplied alcohol so that lighter drinkers had to pay more for their drink. However, because the new price was less than the previous black market prices, moderate and heavy drinkers found that their drinks were cheaper. In consequence, when rationing was stopped the greatest increases in consumption were seen in those who had been heavy consumers when rationing was in force.

It is difficult, given the important effects of price and public opinion, to measure the effect on consumption of retail availability, although such an analysis has been done.[15] There is no doubt that such an effect does exist and careful consideration should be given to any decision that increases the number of retail alcohol outlets.

## ▶ Control of opening hours – the Scottish experience

In 1976, as a response to some of the recommendations of the Clayson report,[16] some relaxation of the licensing law was permitted in Scotland. Opening hours were extended from 10 pm to 11 pm; Sunday opening times were introduced; some 24-hour licences were allowed. The effects of these changes (which are, in proportional terms, fairly minor) have since been hotly debated.

A survey of drinking habits was conducted in 1984, and comparisons were made with the results of a survey carried out immediately prior to the licensing changes.[17] A 13 per cent increase in consumption per head of adult population was discovered, although this did not reach statistical significance at the 5 per cent level. Most of this increase was due to changes in consumption by women, in whom an increased frequency of drinking occasions, and an increase in the proportion who drank was noted.

In 1986 J. Duffy and M. Plant reviewed several indicators of consumption levels, including mortality from liver cirrhosis, mortality due to alcohol dependence, drink-driving convictions, and first admissions to psychiatric wards for alcohol psychoses.[18] The authors observed that alcohol-related harm had been increasing throughout the 1970s, and that the rates did not vary much in relation to those of England and Wales. They concluded that the effects of the change in the law were neutral. However, the authors took no account of policing attitudes in the run-up to the changes in the law, which may have altered in the light of anticipated relaxation. Other criticisms were made, in particular that the data analysed were too soft to detect the effect of these legal changes.[19]

The changes wrought by altered licensing laws may have subtle effects on the patterns of drinking which are not detected by trends in overall consumption or alcohol-related harm. It has been claimed that the Scottish changes led to more sensible drinking habits, although this has been disputed by P. Davies who warns that too little is known about the effects of such changes on the distribution of consumption for such conclusions to be drawn.[20] Nevertheless, a trend towards a reduced rate of consumption was detected in Scotland, although it was not statistically significant.[21] In 1984, an increased proportion of overall drinking took place in pubs and private homes instead of hotels and clubs, due mainly to changes in the drinking habits of all women and of heavily drinking males.

A study of overdoses in Scotland compared experience in the five years after the changes in licensing law with experience in the five years before. Among men there was a 23 per cent increase in the proportion of overdoses associated with alcohol, while in women there was a 21 per cent increase. This study also demonstrated a sharp increase in total admissions for overdose after the law change in 1976.[22]

The restriction of opening hours is, from experience of the Scottish changes, an effective influence upon the level of alcohol consumption. Attempts to engineer change in social habits of drinking by altering licence controls may have unexpected, subtle effects upon the distribution of alcohol consumption among the population.

The licensing laws were amended in England and Wales in 1988. These amendments provided for extended opening hours but also allowed the Licensing Justices greater powers to restrict or revoke licenses. A preliminary survey was conducted and will be repeated in order to assess the effect of those changes on the drinking habits of the population.[23]

## ▶ The age limit

The prohibition of drinking below a certain age can be effective. As with all laws, the degree of that effect depends entirely upon the degree to which it is enforced. When the legal age for alcohol purchase was raised in New York, reported alcohol purchasing by eighteen-year-olds as assessed by telephone survey was found to have fallen and this effect persisted for at least three years.[24] The telephone survey is a method which is open to criticism, as telephone owners may be unrepresentative and more likely to comply with legal restrictions than non-telephone owners. It is difficult to know whether the reduction was real, or was the result of not wishing to confess to crime.

A more robust assessment of the effect of age limitation was made in Australia where three states lowered the legal age for drinking from twenty-one to eighteen in the early 1970s.[25] Male juvenile (age 17–21) crime showed a 20–25 per cent increase when compared with juvenile crime in states which did not alter their legislation, or with juvenile crime in the three states before they reduced the legal age. This increase was not consistent in type across the three states. Only a slight increase was seen for girls. There was also an increase in traffic accident casualties associated with the lowering of the minimum drinking age.[26] The authors concluded that a twenty or twenty-one age limit is to be preferred to one of eighteen and many American States would agree with this conclusion,

A large proportion of crime is committed by juveniles, and much of it is alcohol-related. The problems of drinking and driving are exacerbated by youth. The legal minimum age for alcohol consumption should be more rigorously enforced and consideration should be given to banning young adults from drinking before driving.

## ▶ Changing sales patterns

The availability of alcohol is an important, although not independent, factor in the overall consumption of alcohol. Within that overall consumption, the pattern of access to alcohol has a significant effect on the pattern of consumption.

The Clayson report,[27] for example, sought to relax licensing laws, to introduce families into the drinking environment, and so create the licensed café shops of France which, it was felt, would limit the worst excesses of drunkenness. But there is some concern that this change might increase consumption in the UK towards the much higher levels seen in France. This change might be accompanied by an increase in cirrhosis rates towards the much higher (five times) rates seen in France.[28]

Important changes are occurring in our society, as cheaper foreign travel allows increasing exposure to foreign and unfamiliar patterns of alcohol availability, and as the increasingly unified Common Market urges a more uniform social culture. Already, exposure of this country's youth to readily available alcohol abroad has contributed to an unpopular public image of drunkenness and aggression.

In recent decades, the pattern of alcohol sales in this country has been changing significantly. For most of this century, alcohol consumption was a male-dominated habit, centred in male-orientated licensed premises. More recently, there has been an increasing amount of alcohol being consumed away from the point of purchase[29] as well as an increase in the proportion of heavy drinkers amongst women, despite the lack of a similar increase amongst men.[30,31] These changes are reflected by changes in marketing practice. Over the ten years to 1987, the number of off-licence premises increased by 30 per cent, whereas licensed premises increased by only 15 per cent. In 1987, 25 per cent of the total retail drink turnover was through off-licence premises compared with 20 per cent in 1972.[32]

The increasing importance to the market of women shoppers is reflected by the decline of specialist alcohol shops (seen by the trade as male-orientated outlets) relative to grocers and super-markets (seen as female-orientated), with the latter taking more than 50 per cent of the off-licence trade for the first time in 1987.[33,34] The pattern of drinking also shows this change in habit; since 1980, the overall consumption of beer has fallen, while that of spirits has remained steady and the consumption of wines has increased dramatically (see Figure 5.1). From 1960 to 1981, the consumption of wine (in litres per capita of population aged over 14 years) increased more than five times, while that of spirits more than doubled. In the same period, the consumption of beer increased by less than one half (see Figure 5.2). When one

FIGURE 5.1    *Trends in consumption of alcoholic drinks 1980–87*

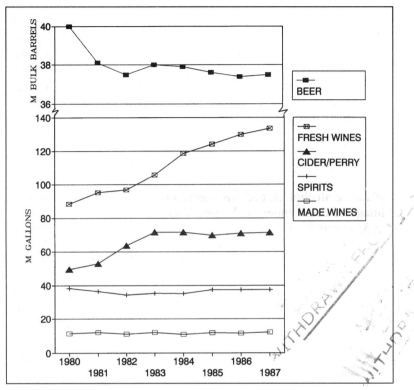

Figures for spirits are shown in proof gallons.

SOURCE    Customs and Excise figures

considers that the percentage of total sales conducted through off licence premises is 13.4 per cent for beer, 19 per cent for lager, 68 per cent for spirits, 73 per cent for still wines and 87 per cent for fortified wines,[35] it is clear that those drink types of which consumption is most rapidly increasing are also those which are sold mostly through off-licence outlets.

It is difficult to say whether the changing pattern of retail sales followed or led the public demand for increasing off-licence purchases and more drinking by women. Whichever is the case, licensing restrictions are capable of limiting any such expansion of the market and consequent increase in alcohol consumption.

FIGURE 5.2    *Changes in consumption, 1960 and 1981*

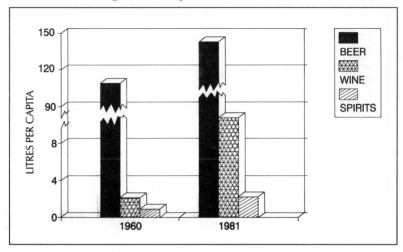

SOURCE    B. Walsh and M. Grant, *Public health implications of alcohol production and trade*, WHO Offset Publication No. 88 (Geneva: WHO, 1985).

## ▶ Licensing Justices

The duty of the Government is to provide a legislative framework within which local communities might regulate, by licence, public availability of alcohol. Some issues which have been discussed above (such as the lower age limit for purchasing alcohol) may be determined only by the national government. Others are largely controlled by the actions of the local Licensing Justices.

Licensing Justices act under the provision of the Licensing Act of 1964, which has since been amended on several occasions. A guide to the licensing laws is available.[36] The Licensing Justice is a magistrate, appointed by his peers, who operates by holding regular licensing sessions. There must be at least four licensing sessions in any one year and one general annual licensing meeting which is held in February (the Brewster Sessions). Two major types of licence are given. On-licences permit the sale of alcohol for consumption on or off the premises (special licences exist for restaurants and residential institutions). Off-licences may sell alcohol only for consumption off the premises. Wholesale outlets (where the minimum quantity of purchase is nine litres of wine or spirits, or twenty-one litres of beer or cider) do not require a licence.

Justices may under Section 3(1) of the Licensing Act 1964 grant a licence to any person they judge suitable regardless of any notion of 'need' or 'demand', although Justices usually do require evidence of such need. Refusal of a licence may be challenged by appeal to the Crown Court.

## ▶ Licensing policies

Insufficient attention is paid by some Licensing Justices to the wider implications of their decisions for alcohol consumption and alcohol-related harm in the community. The legal requirement that every application for a licence be considered on its own merits, and not in the light of an overall strategy of licensing for the relevant area, may have deterred some Benches from considering the wider implications of their decisions.

Most areas do not have a written licensing policy but a small minority have produced such policies. A model licensing policy is being drawn up by the Justices' Clerks Society. This is included as an Appendix in P. Tether and D. Robinson.[37] The current secretary to the Justices' Clerks Society is Mr. A. Heath, The Court House, Homer Road, Solihull B91 3RD. The model policy already mentioned demonstrates that an overall framework of concern is not incompatible with a case-by-case appraisal of applications. The Justices' Clerks' Society identifies five factors which are described as the 'overriding considerations' for each case. These are considerations of (a) Public safety; (b) Public order; (c) Public nuisance; (d) Likelihood of non–compliance with the law; and (e) Local levels of alcohol abuse.

There is no doubt that public disorder and nuisance are related to the availability of alcohol through retail purchase. However, it is equally certain that these problems are also related to the policies by which the licensing laws are administered and enforced.

Licensing forums will be discussed in Chapter 9.

*Recommendation No. 14*

It is recommended that every licensing authority adopts and produces a clear written statement of licensing policy.

## ► Police and the Licensing Justices

It is already a requirement of law that the police authorities submit an annual report to the relevant Licensing Justice. The police also process new applications, investigate the suitability of the applicant and the quality of the premises. Not every police force has either a department responsible for these duties, or an interest in preventive policing of licensed premises.

Licensing Justices should satisfy themselves that the police have sufficient resources and commitment to enforce the law. The results of the police surveillance activity should be a part of the annual report made by the police to the Licensing Justices who would be able to take the observations made into account when making decisions on subsequent applications.

*Recommendation No. 15*

It is recommended that, as with Licensing Justices' policies, every police authority should have a written statement of intent regarding surveillance of licensed premises and preventive policing of those areas identifiable as likely to give rise to alcohol-related problems.

## ► The concept of need for a new licence

Licensing Justices are not required to consider the 'need' for any new licence, although they generally do so. The concept of 'need' is difficult to understand when related to a product which, although associated with some social benefits, is not necessary to society and may be the cause of great harm. In an overall legislative framework which permits the availability of alcohol, it is difficult for a Licensing Justice to counter an argument of commercial logic which states that there is a consumer demand for a particular licence in any one area. For a Licensing Justice to deny an application on the grounds of no need is to open themselves to subsequent reversal upon appeal to a Crown Court.

> *Recommendation No. 16*
>
> It is recommended that the law should require the Licensing Justice to balance the commercial demand for such a licence against current levels of provision within an area, and against the risk that such a licence poses to Public Order, Safety and Health.

## ▶ Control at the point of sale

In view of the trend towards drinking away from the point of purchase, it is important to note the differences in control at point of sale. The licensee for on-premises drinking is under legal obligation not to sell alcohol to an inebriated person, although this law is not widely enforced. They are also responsible for ensuring reasonable standards of behaviour while drinkers are on their premises. The importance of the drinking environment will be discussed in Chapter 10.

There is less opportunity for such direct control of drunkenness through off-license premises, however. People cannot be prevented from buying large quantities of alcohol, with the intention of consuming it later in a public place, and then behaving in a drunken and sometimes violent fashion.

Alcohol should continue to be regarded as a 'special' goods. It is a drug which should not become part of regular grocery sales, even if under 'shop within a shop' arrangements, by which the alcohol must be bought at a counter separate from those used for other goods. Licensing Justices should ensure that adequate arrangements are made to prevent pilfering of alcohol, and to prevent sales to customers who are under the legal minimum age. These requirements are more difficult to ensure in a large supermarket than in a specialist alcohol outlet.

It is of crucial importance that drinking and driving be seen as incompatible activities. The 1988 Licensing Act disqualified premises used primarily as a garage from receiving a licence. However premises licensed prior to 22 August 1988 can retain and renew their licences provided that they have not been allowed to lapse. Drinking and any form of work with moving machinery are also incompatible, so due consideration should be given to the problems that might arise from licensed premises at places of work.

The control of alcohol sales has an important part to play in controlling consumption and the related harm. Licensing Justices should be aware of the full extent of their influence in this regard, and should be fully cognisant of the overall picture, within which they are making decisions that directly concern the welfare of the local community. There should be full and informed liaison between police, magistrates and the caring agencies.

## ▶ Drinking in public places

There has always been concern about drunken behaviour in public places and the spate of publicity given to 'lager louts' is one more manifestation of this anxiety. Drinking was believed to contribute to the violence and public disorder which occurred at football matches and the Government responded by banning alcohol sales in football grounds and on designated trains used by football supporters.

There was also public anxiety over drunken behaviour by people drinking in public areas in the centre of towns or cities. Six councils have now introduced bye-laws which within designated areas make it an offence to consume alcoholic drink in a public place and continue to do so after having been requested to stop by a police constable. One city with such a bye-law is Coventry and it is notable that there were no arrests on carnival day after the law was introduced, whereas in previous years there had been 30–60 arrests. Surveys of residents show the new bye-law to be generally popular.[38]

References

1. C. Clayson, *Report of the departmental committee on Scottish licensing law* (London: HMSO, 1972).

2. Errol of Hale, *Report of the departmental committee on liquor licensing* (London: HMSO, 1971).
3. DHSS, *Advisory Committee on Alcoholism: Report on Prevention* (London: HMSO, 1978).
4. WHO, *Problems related to alcohol consumption*, Technical Report Series 650 (Geneva: WHO, 1980).
5. B. Jeffs and W. Saunders, 'Minimising alcohol-related offences by enforcement of the existing licensing legislation', *British Journal of Addiction*, 78(1983) pp. 67–77.
6. I. Wald and J. Moskalewicz, 'Alcohol Policy in a crisis situation', *British Journal of Addiction*, 79(1984) pp. 331–5.
7. Royal College of Psychiatrists, *Alcohol – our favourite drug* (London: Tavistock, 1986).
8. E. Osterberg, *Recorded consumption of alcohol in Finland 1950–1975* (Helsinki: Social Research Institute of Alcohol Studies, 1982).
9. T. McGuinness, 'An econometric analysis of total demand for alcoholic beverages in the United Kingdom 1956–1975', *Journal of Industrial Economics*, 39(1980) pp. 85–109.
10. R. E. Popham, W. Schmidt and L. de Lint, 'The prevention of Alcoholism: epidemiological studies of the effects of government control measures', *British Journal of Addiction*, 70(1975) pp. 125–44.
11. H. Holder and J. Blose, 'Impact of changes in distilled spirits availability on apparent consumption; a time series analysis of liquor by the drink', *British Journal of Addiction*, 82(1987) pp. 623–31.
12. J. Blose and H. Holder, 'Liquor by the drink and alcohol-related crashes: a natural experiment using time series analyses', *Journal of Studies of Alcohol*, 78(1987) pp. 52–6.
13. R. Smart, 'The effect of licensing restrictions during 1914–1918 on drunkenness and liver cirrhosis deaths in Britain', *British Journal of Addiction*, 69(1974) pp. 109–21.
14. T. Norstrom, 'The abolition of the Swedish Alcohol Rationing System: effects on consumption, distribution and cirrhosis mortality', *British Journal of Addiction*, 82(1987) pp. 633–41.
15. T. McGuiness, 'An econometric analysis of total demand for alcoholic beverages in the UK', op. cit.
16. C. Clayson, *Report on Scottish licensing laws*, op. cit.
17. E. L. Goddard, *Drinking and attitudes to licensing in Scotland in 1984* (London: HMSO, 1988).
18. J. Duffy and M. Plant, 'Scotland's liquor licensing laws: an assessment', *British Medical Journal*, 292(1986) pp. 36–9.
19. J. Eagles and J. Besson, 'Scotland's liquor licensing changes', *British Medical Journal*, 292(1986) p. 486.
20. P. Davies, 'The Licensing (Scotland) Act 1976', *British Journal of Addiction*, 83(1988) pp. 129–30.

21. E. L. Goddard, *Drinking and attitudes to licensing in Scotland*, op. cit.
22. D. Northridge, J. McMurray and A. Lawson, 'Association between liberalisation of Scotland's liquor licensing laws and admissions for self poisoning in West Fife', *British Medical Journal*, 293(1986) pp. 1466–8.
23. E. Goddard and C. Ikin, *Drinking in England and Wales in 1987* (London: HMSO, 1988)).
24. T. Williams and R. Lillis, 'Long-term changes in reported alcohol purchasing and consumption following an increase in New York State's purchasing age to 19', *British Journal of Addiction*, 83(1988) pp. 209–17.
25. D. Smith and P. Burvill, 'Effect on juvenile crime of lowering the drinking age in three Australian States', *British Journal of Addiction*, 82(1987) pp. 181–8.
26. R. Smart and M. Goodstadt, 'Effects of reducing the legal alcohol purchasing age on drink driving problems', *Journal of Studies of Alcohol*, 38(1977) pp. 1313–23.
27. C. Clayson, op. cit.
28. Office of Health Economics, *Alcohol: Reducing the Harm* (London: Office of Health Economics, 1981).
29. *The Drinks Market Profile*, Stats MR/Off Licence news (London: William Reed, 1988).
30. Royal College of General Practitioners, *Alcohol – a balanced view*. Reports from General Practice 24 (London: Royal College of General Practitioners, 1986).
31. P. Wilson, *Drinking in England and Wales* (OPCS) (London: HMSO, 1980).
32. *The Drinks Market Profile*, op. cit.
33. Ibid.
34. *The Take Home Market* (Off Licence News) (London: William Reed, 1988).
35. *The Drinks Market Profile*, op. cit.
36. M. Underhill, *A Licensing Guide*, 10th ed. (London: Longman, 1989).
37. P. Tether and D. Robinson, *Preventing Alcohol Problems: A guide to local action* (London: Tavistock, 1986).
38. M. Ramsay, *Downtown drinkers*. Home Office Crime Prevention paper 19. (London: Home Office, 1989).

# ▶6▶ ▶ ▶ ▶ ▶ ▶ ▶ ▶ ▶ ▶ ▶ ▶ ▶ ▶

# DOES TAXATION AFFECT CONSUMPTION?

The previous chapter considered the possibility of controlling mean alcohol consumption, frequency of heavy consumption and the frequency of alcohol-related harm by regulating the times, places and conditions under which alcohol could be sold. This chapter considers the possibility of influencing alcohol consumption by manipulating price through taxation.

## ▶ Relative price and consumption

There appears to be a strong relationship between the amount of alcohol consumed and the price relative to income. Figure 6.1 shows how the consumption of alcohol in the UK increased as its relative price fell, and Figure 6.2 shows similar data for Ontario.[1]

The amount of work time required to earn the price of a pint of draught beer and a bottle of whisky for a male manual worker is shown in Figure 6.3. A male manual worker had to work less than half the amount of time in 1974 than he did in 1964 to purchase a bottle of whisky, and a quarter less time for a pint of beer. Since 1974, work effort required has declined less rapidly for the purchase of a bottle of whisky, but risen for a pint of beer.[2]

## ▶ Effect of price versus income

Relative price is affected by changes in price and changes in income, but a fall in price and a rise in income may not have the

FIGURE 6.1   *Relation of relative price of alcohol and alcohol consumption*

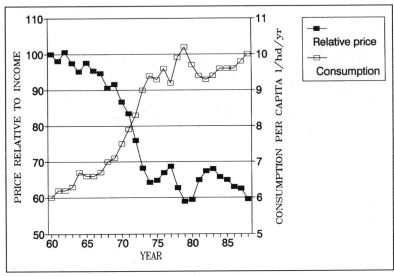

Relative price is price relative to income (1960 = 100).

Consumption shown in litres of alcohol per head of population aged 15 or over.

SOURCE   C. Godfrey (personal communication).

same effect on consumption. The level of income or purchasing power can affect consumption of alcohol independently of price.[3]

It is possible to dissociate the effect of price and income by a technique known as time series regression analysis. This procedure examines the relationship between income, price and consumption and quantifies the income and price elasticities of demand for alcoholic products.[4] The price elasticity of demand is a measure of the change of the demand for a product when its price changes. The income elasticity of demand is a measure of the change in the demand for a product when the income of consumers changes.

A report by the United Kingdom Treasury[5] suggests that for a 1 per cent rise in the real price of alcohol consumer demand for beer might be expected to fall by about 0.25 per cent, for spirits by about 1.5 per cent, and for wine, by about 1 per cent. However, a 1 per cent rise in real incomes might be expected to

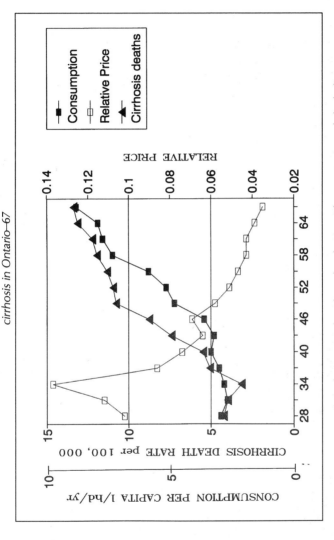

FIGURE 6.2    *Consumption of alcohol, relative price of alcohol and deaths from liver cirrhosis in Ontario–67*

SOURCE    R. E. Popham, W. Schmidt and L. de Lint, The prevention of alcoholism, *British Journal of Addition*, 70 (1975) pp. 125–44

FIGURE 6.3  *Time that a male manual worker needs to work to earn the price of a pint of beer or the price of a bottle of whisky*

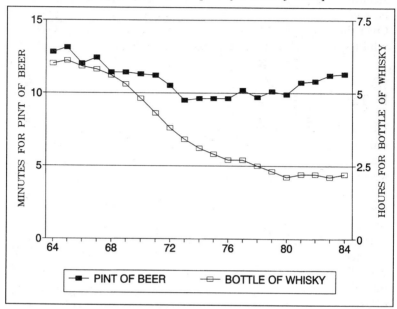

SOURCE  C. Godfrey, G. Hardman and M. Powell, 'Alcohol, Tobacco and Taxation', *British Journal of Addiction*, 81(1986) pp. 143–9.

increase consumer demand for beer by about 0.75 per cent, for spirits by about 2.25 per cent, and for wine by about 2.5 per cent. This suggests that over the years consumption of beer, the predominant alcoholic beverage in the United Kingdom, has been less sensitive to changes in price and income than wines and spirits. It also suggests that consumption of alcoholic drinks is less sensitive to rises in price than it is to rises in disposable income.

## ▶ Effect of tax on price

Taxation can be used as an instrument to vary the price of alcoholic drinks. Currently excise duty accounts for about 60 per cent of the retail price of spirits, 40 per cent of the retail price of beer and 40 per cent of the retail price of wine. Changes in duty therefore have a considerable influence on the retail cost of alcohol. The effects of recent budgetary adjustments in duty can be seen in the price changes of alcohol presented in Table 6.1. Over the time period beer has become relatively more expensive, whilst spirits and wine have become considerably cheaper.[6]

## ▶ Taxes on Alcohol

During the last twenty years alcohol taxation has undergone a number of structural changes. Prior to 1973 alcohol excise duties were levied at different rates on different types of alcoholic beverage. In 1973 a general VAT (Value Added Tax) component was added to these alcohol excise duties at a rate initially set at 8 per cent but increasing to 15 per cent by 1979. The current levels of alcohol excise duties for different types of alcohol and different strengths are shown in the last line of Table 6.1.

Since 1979, Chancellors of the Exchequer have stated that general budget policy is to increase excise duties in line with inflation (revalorisation). There have, however, been a number of exceptions.[7] The most striking exception is the fall in the value of duty on wine in the 1984 Budget. This move was a necessary response to a European Court ruling in 1983 suggesting that the UK overtaxed wine relative to beer. The Court ruled that wine and beer should be taxed at similar rates according to strength per volume. Another exception to the overall strategy of inflation-proofing is shown by the year-to-year variation in the level of taxation on spirits. In 1985, the Chancellor cited the problems of the Scotch whisky industry to justify a tax increase of less than half the rate of inflation.

## ▶ Objectives and constraints of alcohol taxation policy

The government may have a number of objectives when determining its alcohol taxation policy:[8, 9]

1. Generation of revenue
2. Fostering employment and local manufacture
3. Controlling cost of living and inflation
4. Limitation of harmful effects of alcohol consumption

TABLE 6.1 Excise duty on alcohol, 1980–90

| Date | Duty on spirits | | Duty on beer | | Duty on wine | |
|---|---|---|---|---|---|---|
| | Duty per litre of alcohol | Estimated price effect of duty change on bottle of whisky | Duty per hectolitre at 10.30° | Estimated price effect of duty change on pint of beer | Duty per hectolitre 15°–18° | Estimated price effect of duty change on bottle of table wine |
| | £ | p | £ | p | £ | p |
| March 1980 | 11.87 | 50 | 13.05 | 2 | 93.93 | 8 |
| March 1981 | 13.60 | 60 | 18.00 | 4 | 112.90 | 12 |
| March 1982 | 14.47 | 30 | 20.40 | 2 | 137.90 | 10 |
| March 1983 | 15.19 | 25 | 21.60 | 1 | 145.90 | 5 |
| March 1984 | 15.48 | 10 | 24.00 | 2 | 157.50 | 18 |
| March 1985 | 15.77 | 10 | 25.80 | 1 | 169.00 | 10 |
| March 1986 | 15.77 | 0 | 25.80 | 0 | 169.00 | 0 |
| March 1987 | 15.77 | 0 | 25.80 | 0 | 169.00 | 0 |
| March 1988 | 15.77 | 0 | 27.00 | 1 | 176.60 | 4 |
| March 1989 | 15.77 | 0 | 27.00 | 0 | 176.60 | 0 |
| March 1990 | 17.35 | 54 | 29.10 | 2 | 190.22 | 7 |

SOURCES  C. Godfrey and M. Powell, *Budget strategies for alcohol and tobacco tax in 1987 and beyond*. Discussion Paper 22 (York: Centre for Health Economics, 1987); and for 1987 onwards Budget Statements.

# ▶ Tax revenue and alcohol

Taxes on alcohol are an important source of Government revenue (see Figure 6.4). Real tax yields were higher in 1985 than in 1979 despite a fall in the share of alcohol in total revenue. In 1979, excise and VAT on beer constituted 43 per cent of alcohol revenue, spirits 41 per cent and wines just 16 per cent. By 1985, wine revenue increased to 19 per cent of alcohol revenue, beer to 50 per cent and spirits declined to 31 per cent. These changes reflect changes in both consumption patterns and tax policy.[10]

Alcohol tax offers many advantages to Government because it is a relatively cheap and easy tax to collect and causes little market distortion. Because the demand for alcohol is price inelastic, a one per cent rise in its price results in a less than

FIGURE 6.4   *Revenue from taxation on alcoholic drink*

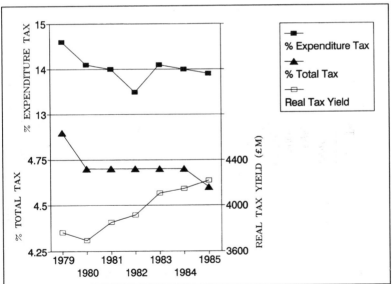

Real tax yields (adjusted to 1980 prices) for alcohol taxation are shown. Alcohol taxation is also shown as a percentage of revenue from taxes on expenditure and as a percentage of total tax revenue.

SOURCE   As Figure 6.3

one per cent fall in consumption. Thus when tax is levied on alcohol, the level of substitution for other products is low and the effect on revenue earned of any decline in consumption is more than offset by the increased revenue from the remainder. Excise tax on alcohol is therefore part of general revenue policy.[11]

## ▶ Trade, industry and employment

Excise policy is likely to be influenced by balance of trade considerations as well as domestic production trends. Recent trends in consumption, trade and employment in the alcohol industry are shown in Figure 6.5. Spirits exports and wine imports dominate the trade in alcohol. In general, the UK has been a net exporter of alcohol in value terms but in recent years the balance is shifting to a less favourable position reflecting an increase in both beer and wine imports.[12]

Consumption of alcohol fell during the recession years of 1980–82. Figure 6.5 shows that this was accompanied by a 10 per cent fall in the numbers employed in the alcohol industry but when consumption increased again the numbers employed continued to fall. The Government has declared a policy of protection for the spirits industry. However, total consumption of beer has fallen (being 10 per cent lower in 1985 than 1979) and the Government is likely to take the effects of tax policy on domestic beer producers into account.

## ▶ Inflation

Levels of inflation are also taken into consideration for tax policy on alcohol. Changes in excise tax have a direct effect on the rate of price changes in the economy but the effects are small. A revalorisation of all excise duties, including petrol, derv (fuel oil for heavy vehicles) and vehicle duty, in March 1987 of 3.25 per cent only raised the Retail Price Index by 0.3 per cent.[13] The desirability of including alcoholic drinks in the Retail Price Index used for the calculation of inflation is discussed later.

FIGURE 6.5    *Recent trends in expenditure on alcohol (adjusted to 1980 prices)*

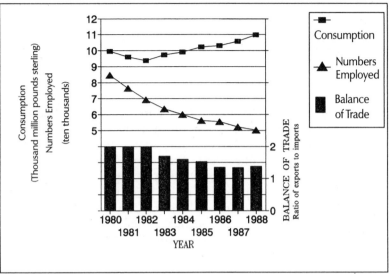

Consumption in thousand million pounds value terms (adjusted to 1980 prices).
Numbers (ten thousands) directly employed in alcohol trade.
Balance of Trade (ratio of alcohol export to imports in value terms).

SOURCES    Consumption and balance of trade: as Figure 6.3. Numbers employed: from C. Godfrey and K. Hartley, Data note 16 Employment and prevention policy, *British Journal of Addiction*, 83(1988) pp. 1335–42, with additional data from Godfrey (personal communication).

## ▶ Payment of indirect social costs

The costs of alcohol consumption can be divided into internal and external. Internal costs are the costs of raw materials, labour to make the product, transport, advertising, stockholding and retailing. External costs are the unmarketable and unwanted costs imposed on third parties by some drinkers, such as from drinking and driving, or from the psychological and physical distress imposed on family and friends. An indirect excise tax can target these external costs of consumption on the consumer thereby improving market efficiency.[14, 15]

## ▶ Alcohol tax as a prevention policy

The Government may choose to use alcohol taxation as a component of a policy intended to reduce alcohol-related harm.[16] Alcohol is taxed with the deliberate intention of discouraging the purchase of the product. Government may choose to implement this type of policy on the basis of improving the market mechanisms and raising welfare, or on the basis of altering the value drinkers place on their actions.

Once it is accepted that one of the purposes of alcohol taxation could be to influence consumption of alcohol there is a logical basis for tax banding. Rates of duty should be adjusted so that they reflect the alcohol content of the drink. The likely effects of these changes has been explored using econometric models.[17, 18]

Some low-alcohol products are at present taxed at the same rate as normal strength products since duty is assessed on the alcohol content at an intermediate stage of the production process, and not of the final product. This anomaly is a disincentive to responsible drinking and should be ended.

*Recommendation No. 17*

It is recommended that the Government should deliberately adopt a policy of taxing alcoholic drinks so as to reduce consumption. At the very least alcohol prices should not be allowed to fall and should be revalorised for changes in price and then further revalorised for changes in income.

*Recommendation No. 18*

It is recommended that duties should be based on the alcohol content of the drink. Duty on different drink types should be adjusted so that the duty on one unit of alcohol is similar for all drink types. Tax bandings within each drink type should be adjusted so that proportionately more duty is payable on drinks of higher alcohol content.

> *Recommendation No. 19*
>
> It is recommended that duty should be based on the alcohol content of the final product and that no duty should be payable on alcohol-free products regardless of their method of manufacture. (Recent changes have met this recommendation.)

## ▶ The European Community

The freedom of many European countries to fix taxation levels for alcoholic drinks is circumscribed by the Treaty of Rome. The European Community is seeking to create a Common Market in all goods including alcoholic drinks by removing internal barriers to trade, and is seeking to harmonise tax levels so that products are treated equally by the tax system of the ten member countries. Because the UK has higher taxation on alcohol (especially wine) than most other member states the likely effect of harmonisation will be to oblige the United Kingdom to reduce taxation on wine and thereby reduce the price.[19, 20]

Harmonisation could be achieved in several different ways. Under the proposals in the Cockfield Report,[21] duty on all alcoholic drinks would be reduced, with the greatest reduction in duty on wine and least reduction in duty on spirits (see Figure 6.6). The estimated effect of this change would be to increase alcohol consumption in the United Kingdom by 46 per cent and to more than double the numbers of those consuming more than 50 units per week.[22] Such a change in consumption would be expected to significantly increase the frequency of alcohol-related problems. Other ways of achieving harmonisation would have a less severe effect on consumption.

> *Recommendation No. 20*
>
> It is recommended that the Government should negotiate with a view to ensuring that harmonisation of tariffs in 1992 does not result in a significant reduction in the price of alcoholic drinks in the UK.

FIGURE 6.6    *Effect on alcohol taxation of indirect taxes within European market — effect of Cockfield proposals*

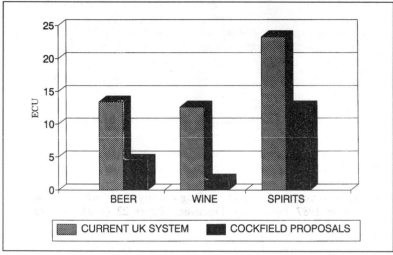

SOURCE    P. Baker and S. McKay, *The Structure of Alcohol Taxes: A Hangover from the Past?*, IFS Commentary No. 21 (London: Institute for Fiscal Studies, 1990), figure 2. Reproduced by kind permission of the Institute of Fiscal Studies.

## ▶ Alcohol in the Retail Price Index

The Retail Price Index is based on the prices of a notional shopping basket which includes cigarettes and alcohol. The inclusion of alcohol is undesirable, not only because it implies that alcohol is an indispensable part of living but also because it discourages Chancellors from using alcohol taxation as a device for the prevention of alcohol-related harm. The minor cosmetic change of removing alcohol from the Retail Price Index would make it easier to implement a tax policy which promoted public health.

*Recommendation No. 21*

It is recommended that the basis on which the Retail Price Index is calculated should be amended so as to exclude alcohol.

References

1. R. E. Popham, W. Schmidt and L. de Lint, 'The prevention of alcoholism: epidemiological studies of the effects of government control measures', *British Journal of Addiction*, 70(1975) pp. 125–44.
2. C. Godfrey, G. Hardman and M. Powell, 'Alcohol, Tobacco and Taxation', *British Journal of Addiction*, 81(1986) pp. 143–9.
3. T. McGuinness, 'An econometric analysis of total demand for alcoholic beverages in the UK, 1956–75', *Journal of Industrial Economics*, September 1980, pp. 85–109.
4. C. Godfrey, *Factors influencing the consumption of alcohol and tobacco – a review of demand models.* Discussion Paper 17 (York: Centre for Health Economics, 1986).
5. HM Treasury, *Macroeconomic Model Equation and Variable Listing* (London: HM Treasury, 1986).
6. C. Godfrey and M. Powell, *Budget strategies for alcohol and tobacco tax in 1987 and beyond.* Discussion Paper 22 (York: Centre for Health Economics, 1987).
7. C. Godfrey *et al.*, 'Alcohol, Tobacco and Taxation', op. cit.
8. A. Maynard, 'Economic measures in preventing drinking', in N. Heather, I. Robertson and P. Davies (eds) *The Misuse of Alcohol* (London: Croom Helm, 1985).
9. M. Grant, M. Plant and A. Williams, *Economics and Alcohol* (London: Croom Helm, 1982).
10. C. Godfrey and M. Powell, *Budget Strategies*, op. cit.
11. Ibid.
12. C. Godfrey *et al.*, 'Alcohol, Tobacco and Taxation', op. cit.
13. C. Godfrey and M. Powell, *Budget Strategies*, op. cit.
14. M. Grant *et al.*, *Economics and Alcohol*, op. cit.
15. Alcohol Concern, *The Drinking Revolution* (London: Alcohol Concern, 1987).
16. Ibid.
17. E. Crooks, *Alcohol Consumption and Taxation*. Institute for Fiscal Studies Report Series No. 34. (London: Institute for Fiscal Studies, 1989).
18. P. Baker and S. McKay, *The Structure of Alcohol Taxes. A Hangover from the Past*. IFS Commentary No. 21. (London: Institute for Fiscal Studies, 1990).
19. Ibid.
20. A. Maynard and B. O'Brien, 'Harmonisation policies in the European Community and alcohol abuse', *British Journal of Addiction*, 77(1982) pp. 235–44.
21. COM(87) 328 Draft directive on the approximation of rates of excise duty on alcoholic beverages and on the alcohol contained in

other products. Brussels Commission to the European Council (1987).

22.  P. Baker and S. McKay, *The Structure of Alcohol Taxes*, op. cit.

# SEPARATING DRINKING AND DRIVING

Drinking and driving is one of our most serious road safety problems. Alcohol is implicated in approximately 1000 deaths on the road each year, about one in five of all deaths on the road, and one in three of all drivers killed have more than the prescribed limit of alcohol in their blood.[1] At night the proportion rises from one to two-thirds.[2]

## ► Scale of the problem

In 1987 there were 5125 road deaths in Great Britain, 64,000 serious injuries and 242,000 slight injuries as well as many more accidents which go unreported. This represents a major challenge to public health though it is encouraging to note that the toll is less than in earlier years. The number of deaths was 5 per cent lower than in 1986 and the lowest since 1954, while the number of injuries was slightly decreased on the previous year despite an increase in motor traffic.

These figures are taken from the Department of Transport's latest road accident statistics[3] which include only those accidents involving personal injury occurring on the public highway (including footways) in which a road vehicle is involved and which becomes known to the police within thirty days of its occurrence. The vehicle need not be moving and it need not be involved in a collision. One accident may give rise to several casualties.

# ▶ Age distribution of accident victims

Although road accidents represent only 1 per cent of all deaths, the majority of the victims are young, 39 per cent of those killed being under the age of twenty-five. Road accidents represent the single most important cause of death in this age group, accounting for one third of all deaths.[4]

In 1983, 105,000 years of life were lost due to traffic accidents in England and Wales, compared, for example, with 54,000 from lung cancer and 215,000 from coronary heart disease.[5]

# ▶ Alcohol and road traffic accidents

In spite of declining numbers of road traffic casualties there is no room for complacency. It is estimated that at least one in five road traffic accident fatalities were killed in accidents where at least one driver or rider was over the legal blood alcohol limit. It is further estimated that one in ten of non-fatal casualties (25,000 people) sustained their injuries in 'drink-drive' accidents. This figure could well be an underestimate since not all drivers involved in road traffic accidents are breath tested.[6]

The information pointing to a strong association between alcohol and road traffic accidents comes from a variety of indirect sources. Many accident statistics are derived from the accident report forms (known as 'Stats 19') which the police are required to complete for every accident notified to them. Among other things this report records whether the drivers involved in the accident were required to take a breath test and, if so, the result of the test. This source will not identify drink-drive episodes where the driver was unable to give a breath test because he or she was killed or too badly injured, or drink-drive episodes where the accident was not reported.

Coroners in England and Wales and Procurators-fiscal in Scotland supply data to the road research laboratories on blood alcohol levels in individuals aged sixteen or over who die within twelve hours of being injured in a road accident. These statistics complement those derived from the police accident reports.

The number of drivers failing breath tests reaches a maximum around midnight (see Figure 7.1). During the morning period (8.00 am to 11.00 am) only 1 per cent of those tested are positive.

FIGURE 7.1   *Number of positive breath tests at different times of the day*
Note the peak just before midnight

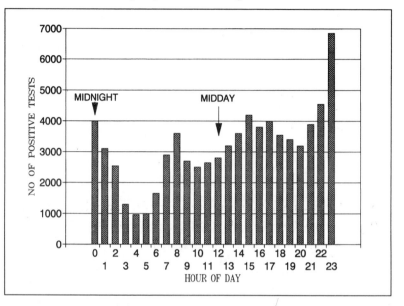

As the day continues the percentage failing the test increases, reaching nearly 9 per cent in the period 3.00 pm to 4.00 pm There is then a small decline in the percentage of tests positive until the start of the 'drink-drive' hours during which time it reaches 33 per cent and remains at 30 per cent between 11.00 pm and 3.00 am.[7] The times when there is a high frequency of positive tests coincide with the times when the risk of accident is high. The number of breath tests carried out by the police has doubled between 1980 and 1987 but the number of positive tests has only increased by one third.

Alcohol-related accidents are more likely to be a single-vehicle accident involving loss of control and excess speed. Since at least one-fifth of road traffic fatalities are definitely associated with alcohol, a large number of these fatalities are potentially preventable, but much needs to be done in order to achieve this reduction. No single course of action will be effective and a number of different approaches including education, training and legislation will be needed to reduce the hazard to road users arising from alcohol.

## ▶ Cost of road traffic accidents

The total cost of road accidents in 1987, including damage only accidents, was estimated at £5 billion. The average cost of a fatal accident was nearly £550,000.[8] It is not possible to give the true costs of road accidents to society, or to compare them directly with the estimated costs of other public health problems, but they represent a major challenge to public health as so many are avoidable.

## ▶ Evidential testing

Alcohol in the blood is measured in milligrams (mg) of alcohol per 100 millilitres (ml) of blood. The legal limit for driving is 80mg per 100ml. The corresponding limit for urine is 107mg/100ml. Alcohol in the breath is measured in micrograms (µg) and the legal limit is 35µg/100ml.

| Equivalents: | Blood | Urine | Breath |
|---|---|---|---|
| | 50mg/100ml | 67mg/100ml | 22µg/100ml |
| Legal limit | 80mg/100ml | 107mg/100ml | 35µg/100ml |
| | 150mg/100ml | 200mg/100ml | 66µg/100ml |
| | 200mg/100ml | 267mg/100ml | 88µg/100ml |
| | 250mg/100ml | 333mg/100ml | 110µg/100ml |

## ▶ The risk of an accident and alcohol levels

Members of the public do not have a clear understanding of the cumulative risk with increasing alcohol intake of being involved in an accident, nor of the way in which alcohol exerts its effect on an individual to cause that increasing risk. It is not generally understood that 80mg/100ml is a *legal* limit for blood alcohol, not a *safe* level.

Although alcohol may give a feeling of well-being its major actions are to interfere with muscular control and co-ordination, lengthen reaction time, blur vision and decrease alertness –

especially in the dark. It also impairs ability to judge speed and distance, and to deal with the unexpected. All these effects adversely affect driving performance. In addition, alcohol impairs judgement, so that many individuals feel increasingly confident in their ability to drive after having consumed alcohol whereas in reality their ability is impaired.

The evidence that alcohol increases the risk of an accident is based on an important controlled study performed in America. This study showed that, compared with someone who has no alcohol in their blood, a driver with blood alcohol level of 80mg/ 100ml is twice as likely to be involved in an accident. At 150mg/ 100ml the risk is increased tenfold and at 200mg/100ml it is increased twentyfold.[9] The risk of accident also varies according to a number of factors such as age, experience of driver and tolerance to alcohol. Inexperienced drivers or those who drink infrequently may be seriously impaired at well below the legal limit (see Figure 7.2).

FIGURE 7.2   *Differences in susceptibility to alcohol*

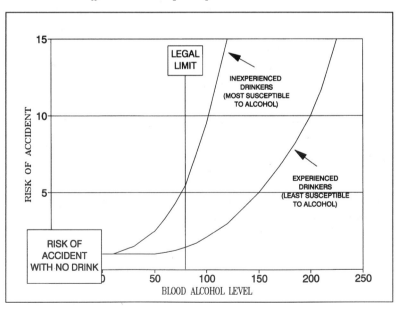

Risk of road accidents at different blood alcohol levels.

## ▶ Factors influencing blood alcohol levels

Although the majority of the general public is now aware of drink-drive legislation there is still a great deal of confusion regarding the alcohol strength of different drinks and the amount needed to produce a blood alcohol level of 80mg/100ml.

There is also a lack of knowledge about the processes by which alcohol is eliminated from the body. The false belief that coffee, food and other substances counteract the effects of alcohol is widely held. The presence of food, particularly fatty food, can slow the absorption of alcohol from the stomach and thus lessen the maximum blood level attained but it cannot affect the rate of elimination. The most rapid absorption into the blood occurs with drinks having about 20 per cent alcohol by volume, such as sherry or gin and tonic, whereas less concentrated drinks such as beer and cider are absorbed more slowly.

Alcohol is eliminated from the body at a rate approximately equivalent to half a pint of beer (normal strength) or a single measure of spirit each hour, that is, one standard unit per hour. If alcohol is consumed at a rate greater than this, it will lead to increasing quantity of alcohol in the body, and hence an increased blood or breath alcohol level. Absorbed alcohol is distributed by the blood and mixes evenly with the water in the body which makes up two-thirds of the body weight. The lighter the person the less water in the body. Therefore, for a given consumption of alcohol, a proportionately higher blood alcohol concentration will be achieved by a lighter person than a heavier individual. Thus women tend to achieve a one-third higher blood alcohol concentration than men for a given consumption of alcohol.

The elimination of alcohol from the body cannot be speeded up. A heavy, late evening drinking session may result in the drinker still being over the legal limit at 7.00 am the next morning. This fact needs to be more widely recognised.

The strength of drinks (for example, normal and strong beers) and the size of drink measures (for example, home measures are often much larger than pub measures) vary widely while individuals have a varying susceptibility to the effects of alcohol. These factors make the estimation of a blood alcohol concentration in any one individual very difficult. This, taken together with the evidence that even small amounts of alcohol can impair performance means the only safe recommendation that can be made to the general public is that if you drink don't drive, and if you are going to drive don't drink.

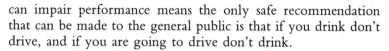

*Recommendation No. 22*

It is recommended that health education should stress that the risk of accident rises with blood alcohol level and that it is substantially increased at levels well below the legal limit. The only safe policy is if you have to drive don't drink alcohol.

## ▶ Drinking pedestrian or drinking driver

Many people do not have the use of a car and others may choose not to use theirs, so the commonest mode of transport for short journeys is walking. In England in 1986 1570 pedestrians (of which 212 were children) were killed in road accidents. The 51,826 pedestrian casualties represented 18 per cent of the total road traffic casualties. Thirty five per cent of the pedestrians killed or injured in road accidents were aged under fifteen and 18 per cent were over sixty.[10] The proportion of total road casualties accounted for by pedestrians has remained roughly constant for the past eight years. The Department of Transport figures exclude pedestrians who were injured in accidents where no vehicle was involved, such as falls in the street (about 200 die in this way each year). If a death occurs following a fall while an individual is trying to avoid a vehicle this would for Department of Transport purposes be classified as a road accident death.

About 400 of the 1400 pedestrian road deaths in 1985 were attributed to drinking by the pedestrian.[11] A pedestrians' risk of suffering a fatal road accident increases with increasing blood alcohol concentrations but is always lower than the risk for a driver with an equivalent level. At very low blood alcohol levels the risk of being involved in an accident for a pedestrian is one-third of that for a vehicle driver with a similar blood alcohol concentration. At blood alcohol levels well above the legal limit the risk of being involved in an accident for a pedestrian is still only half that for a driver.[12] Even if people drink more when they are walking than when they are driving there is a clear benefit in advising people to walk rather than drive after having consumed alcohol.[13]

## ▶ The history of breath testing in the United Kingdom

Breath testing was first introduced by the Road Safety Act 1967 which set the legal limit for driving at 80mg alcohol/100ml of blood. The functioning of the Act was reviewed by the Blennerhassett Committee in 1976 and they produced an important report[14] which is still relevant today. The main recommendations of the Committee were as follows:

(a) The blood/alcohol limit should be retained at 80mg/100ml. (The suggestion that this should be reduced to 50mg/100ml – already debated prior to the 1967 Road Safety Act – was again set aside.)

(b) A constable, at his discretion, should have the power to require a breath test of a person who is or has been driving or attempting to drive or is in charge of a motor vehicle. (It was specifically pointed out that random testing was not intended).

(c) A breath test should normally be used to determine a driver's blood alcohol concentration as well as for roadside screening tests, but with a fallback option of providing blood if the breath analysis is over the limit.

(d) Proof of an offence should not be unreasonably dependent on compliance with procedural requirements.

(e) An order of disqualification for a year (or longer at the court's discretion) should continue to be the main penalty, in conjunction with fines, but in 'high risk' cases (that is, those with very high blood alcohol concentrations, and repeat offenders), licences should not be restored until the court is satisfied that the offender does not present undue risks as a driver.

(f) There should be a continuing programme of publicity, having particular regard to the education of young drivers, to develop informed and responsible attitudes to drinking to enlist public support for the law.

The 1981 Transport Act implemented three of the Blennerhassett proposals (c), (d) and (e). The most recent to be introduced was the roadside Intoximeter (c), which came into effect in 1983.

With reference to recommendation (e), the term 'high risk driver' refers to those disqualified twice in a ten-year period or with a blood/alcohol level two and a half times the legal limit (200mg/100ml) or more. Such offenders will be required to demonstrate that any underlying drink problem has been dealt with before their licence is restored. The introduction of the Intoximeter means that alcohol levels are now measured as microgrammes in 100 millilitres of breath. Offenders have the option of a blood test or, under certain circumstances, a urine test in addition to the Intoximeter reading. The current offences relating to drinking and driving, together with penalties, are defined in the Transport Act 1981.

## ▶ Deterring the drinking driver

The various strategies adopted by the United Kingdom and other countries, and the effectiveness of attempts to deter the drinking driver through law, has been reviewed by L. H. Ross in his book *Deterring the Drinking Driver*.[15] One of the main deterrents to drinking and driving in this country has been the introduction of the breath test. This test has been used in other countries for some years. Its effectiveness is to a large extent dependent on the perceived risk of being apprehended and to a lesser extent by the severity of the penalty meted out following conviction. It is now generally accepted that in the UK only a percentage of drink-drivers are caught and estimates of the chance of being caught whilst driving over the limit range from 1 in 250 to 1 in 4000. The public therefore perceives that there is a low risk of being caught.[16]

## ▶ Breath testing

At the present time, under the Road Safety Act 1967 and the Road Traffic Act 1972, the police may administer a breath test:

(a)  When they suspect that a driver has been drinking;
(b)  When a moving traffic offence has been committed or is suspected;
(c)  When an accident has occurred.

The Road Traffic Act 1972 empowers the police to stop vehicles and they may then decide whether or not there are grounds for requesting a breath test. This has created confusion amongst the general public and there have been accusations of random testing. If the recommendations of the Blennerhassett Committee's Report of 1976 for unfettered discretional testing by the police had been accepted this would have clarified the position. The police would be able to target their activities and stop and test drivers without the reasonable cause to suspect the driver of having consumed alcohol. The deterrent effect would then be increased in line with the perceived chance of being caught.

The two main approaches to widening police powers in breath testing to detect alcohol are:

1.  Unfettered discretional breath testing. This may require a clarification in the law to allow police to request a breath test without providing evidence of reasonable suspicion that a driver had been drinking. The Association of Chief Constables recently recommended that the law should be changed in this way.
2.  Indiscriminate systematic testing. This is popularly referred to as random breath testing. It involves systematically stopping and testing all drivers passing the testing point whether or not they are suspected of drinking and driving.

## ▶ Indiscriminate systematic breath testing

Indiscriminate systematic breath testing would give the police power to set up checkpoints for limited periods (typically half an hour) staffed by between eight and ten policemen, who would test every driver for alcohol using a breath test kit. The success of indiscriminate systematic testing is increased if it is accompanied by publicity campaigns. It must be seen by drivers to be fair, that all are equally likely to be tested and that no particular class of driver or locality is picked on. However, indiscriminate systematic breath testing obviously has manpower implications.

There are, of course, arguments both in favour and against the setting up of indiscriminate systematic breath testing. The arguments in its favour are:

1. It reduces all forms of road accidents by increasing drivers' awareness.
2. To undertake an indiscriminate systematic test takes only a few seconds and therefore causes little delay to drivers. Because of its strong deterrent effect only 0.5 per cent of drivers are likely to be over the limit. The processing of these few will not generally hold up other drivers and will cause minimal delay and inconvenience.
3. Few drivers will face prosecution because of the deterrent effect of indiscriminate systematic testing.
4. The reduction in the numbers of accidents, and thus deaths and injuries, result in a saving to the community and therefore indiscriminate systematic testing is self-financing.
5. The majority of the general population are in favour of indiscriminate systematic breath testing.[17, 18]
6. Indiscriminate systematic testing identifies the problem drinker who is particularly likely to have an accident but is missed by normal policing.[19]

There are a few arguments to be set against the introduction of indiscriminate systematic testing:

1. Impairment of police/public relations. Yet there is no evidence of this occurring in countries such as Australia, New Zealand and Finland, where indiscriminate systematic testing has been adopted.
2. Infringements of civil liberties. This argument was used against the seatbelt legislation, but once this had been implemented over 90 per cent of the population complied and when the legislation was up for review it was passed 'on the nod'.
3. Until recently, the lack of police support and that of some motoring organisations.

*Recommendation No. 23*

It is recommended that police should be given powers to carry out unfettered discretional breath testing. This would empower them to require a breath test without providing evidence of reasonable suspicion that a driver had been drinking.

*Recommendation No. 24*

It is recommended that police should be given powers to conduct indiscriminate systematic breath testing. This would involve stopping all cars passing certain points for limited periods and requiring drivers to give a breath test. This type of testing is often referred to as 'random' testing.

## ▶ Lowering the legal limit

All blood alcohol concentration limits are arbitrary. However, there is good evidence that the risk of being involved in an accident is doubled at levels between 50–60mg/100ml.[20] Therefore some have suggested that lowering the legal limit to 50mg/100ml would reduce the number of road traffic accidents.[21] Many countries such as the Scandinavian countries already have this lower limit and a number have a zero legal limit.[22]

It is estimated that while 1000 deaths and 19,000 injuries could be prevented each year if no driver exceeded the current 80mg/100ml blood alcohol concentration, a further 150 deaths and 6500 injuries could be prevented if no driver exceeded a blood alcohol level of 50mg/100ml. Introduction of a lower 50mg/100ml limit would require a considerable increase in publicity, police enforcement and other deterrent activities.[23] At the present time nearly half of all drink-drive offenders have blood alcohol in excess of 160mg/100ml. It may be argued that police effort would be better spent in enforcing the current 80mg/100ml limit rather than in enforcing lower limits.

## ▶ Zero legal limit

'Zero' legal limit would in fact probably mean a limit of 5mg/100ml because of the legal difficulties in implementing a zero level when an endogenous level (that is, a level resulting from body processes and not from drinking alcohol) could be as high as 2–3mg/100ml. Instrumentation error also needs to be allowed for.

The imposition of a 5mg/100ml limit would enforce the proper view that drinking and driving should be separate activities and that even very small amounts of alcohol in a susceptible individual increases the risk of a road traffic accident. This measure should certainly be considered for provisional licence holders and young drivers who are at an increased risk of being involved in an accident because they are inexperienced at both driving and drinking. It could be argued that these newly qualified drivers should then become a lead cohort of non-drinking drivers.

*Recommendation No. 25*

It is recommended that the legal limit for blood alcohol should be reduced to 50mg/100ml and that further reductions towards the ultimate goal of a 5mg/100ml level should be considered in the future.

## ▶ Organisations campaigning on alcohol and road safety

A number of organisations and groups are currently calling for a reappraisal of both legislation and its implementation to halt the rise in drinking and driving and to act as a greater deterrent.

The Association of Police Surgeons has recently backed a report[24] prepared by Dr James Dunbar, Director of Tayside Safe Driving Project, which includes calls for:

(a) Random breath testing by the police, including saturation enforcement in selected areas.

(b) Reduction of the blood alcohol limit to 50mg – with a limit of 20mg for two years after the granting of a licence to drive.

(c) Abolition of the 'high risk offender' concept in favour of screening all drink-driving offenders and attendance at information/education courses at the offender's expense.

(d) Immediate suspension of the driving licence after a positive test and pending trial.

The Campaign against Drinking and Driving (CADD) is a new pressure group set up in 1985 by two fathers whose children were killed by drunken drivers in two separate accidents.[25] They were dissatisfied with the system of justice which appeared to trivialise the killing of innocent people by drunken drivers. The campaign is to achieve a fairer justice for the victims and says:

(a) Bail should only be allowed on condition that the offender does not drive until the case is heard in court.

(b) Cases to be brought to court much more quickly than at present.

(c) A scaled lowering of blood alcohol levels until a zero level is eventually reached.

(d) A charge of manslaughter to be brought where drunken drivers cause accidents resulting in the deaths of innocent people.

(e) Court cases to be monitored with appropriate protest being made when a sentence appears token or trivial.

(f) Victims be allowed the same rights of appeal as are allowed to the drunken drivers.

Action on Alcohol Abuse established by the Conference of Medical Royal Colleges and their Faculties in the United Kingdom campaigned for:

a. Present blood alcohol level to be retained, but more vigorous enforcement of the law.

b. A zero level for holders of provisional licences and for two years after passing the driving test.

c. Discretionary testing to be introduced.

d. The term 'high risk driver' to be reassessed so as to encompass all offenders.

e.  More involvement of the Probation Service – making attendance at information/education course a condition for probation for second-time offenders.

f.  Information on drinking and driving to be set out more clearly in the Highway Code and knowledge of the matter to be examined as part of the driving test.

The Parliamentary Advisory Council for Transport Safety (PACT) is another organisation which has been set up to campaign for more effective measures. It is an advisory body that looks specifically at the way road safety issues are treated in Parliament.

Alcohol Concern has also launched a campaign, Roadwise, to improve public knowledge regarding the dangers of drinking and driving, and to encourage the development of effective legislation. Road safety organisations and other organisations interested in limiting alcohol-related harm are running similar campaigns.

## ▶ Driving licence withdrawal

Drink-drive offenders do not lose their licences until they have been found guilty by the Court. In 1987 the average time taken to deal with a drink-driving case was 83 days, which allowed plenty of time for the offence to be repeated. The withdrawal of a driving licence pending the case being heard in Court would act as a deterrent.[26]

At the present time the police can only remove a licence from a drinking driver before a case is heard if they proceed by way of arrest, charge and (immediately) produce the accused before a Court. Usually proceedings are adjourned for the prosecution evidence to be prepared and for the defendant to prepare his or her case. A condition of bail can be the prohibition of driving before the trial but this is not often imposed. The vast majority of drink-driving offences are dealt with by the laying of information to a Magistrates Court or Sheriff's District Court at a specific time when the case will be heard.

The North Report[27] advocates the police being prepared to exercise the arrest/charge/production in Court option in appropriate cases thus exploiting the potential of the present Bail

Act 1976 and the Bail Act (Scotland) 1980 more frequently. However, the report emphasises that the measure should be used as an exception and not as a rule, thus not improving the situation a great deal. One predictable drawback of increased stringency over drink-driving offences is that drivers who had been drinking would be tempted to drive on if involved in an accident. This would increase the 'hit and run' rates (failing to stop after an accident).

The law should be strengthened so that all drink-driving offences should result in suspension of the driving licence at the time the offence is detected. This would have an impact on the public attitude and opinion regarding drinking and driving and act as a further deterrent. Withdrawal of the driving licence at the time of the offence before a finding of guilt by a court might be seen as infringing civil liberties. However, in certain circumstances (such as when those accused of an offence are remanded in custody) the requirements of public safety are deemed to override the rights of the individual. The public health interest in immediately taking off the road any driver who drives with blood alcohol levels above 80mg/100ml should take precedence over the interest of those drivers in not losing their licence until they have been brought to Court and convicted.

*Recommendation No. 26*

It is recommended that the law should be amended so that drivers accused of drink-driving offences are prevented from driving in the period between the alleged offence and trial for that offence. The delay before such cases are brought to trial should be minimised.

Some offenders may still drive when disqualified. In one survey published by the Transport and Road Research Laboratory,[28] 10 per cent of drink-drive offenders only had a provisional licence and 11 per cent either had had their licence suspended or had no driving licence. There have been suggestion that driving whilst disqualified should be reclassified as a summary offence, but this proposal should be resisted since it would reduce the deterrent effect of disqualification following conviction for a drink-drive offence.

## ▶ Host liability

It has been suggested that hosts who supply alcohol to drivers who subsequently commit a drink-drive offence should also be liable. The review body in the North Report[29] firmly rejects this possibility of developing criminal/civil 'host liability' legislation for this country – mainly because it would be too difficult to enforce.

However, it suggests that when the Licensing Justices are dealing with the (annual) renewals of licences, they should take into account whether the licensee concerned has regularly appeared to serve drinks to drivers. This would require Magistrates hearing drink-driving cases to enquire where the offender was drinking before being apprehended. Magistrates could ask the police present at a case to ensure that any information as to where the drinking driver was drinking could be passed to the police licensing section and recorded so that it could be produced at renewal time. Alternatively the Clerk to the Justices could institute some kind of record system. Such procedures could be set up on a local basis and thus act as a deterrent to the licensed trade from serving alcohol to a driver who has already had one or two drinks.

*Recommendation No. 27*

It is recommended that the police should enquire of drink-drive offenders where they had been drinking before being apprehended. The names of licensees of premises which had served alcohol to drink-drive offenders should be notified by the police to the Licensing Justices and they should take this information into account when considering the renewal of licences.

## ▶ Hip flask defence

Some drivers caught with increased blood alcohol concentrations following an accident state that their raised blood alcohol concentration was due to having had a drink to reduce their state of shock following the accident. Recent legislation means that this 'hip flask' defence is unlikely to be successful.

## ▶ Insurance schemes

In the past some insurance schemes, such as St Christopher's Insurance Scheme, provided money to pay for a driver following disqualification for a drink-driving offence. Such schemes reduce the deterrent effect of the drink-driving laws. Many drivers are enabled to drink and drive knowing that they will not be seriously affected by disqualification. This is particularly important where a car is essential for work.[30] There is doubt whether these contracts would have been legally enforceable, and following discussion with the Department of Transport, the Association of British Insurers has agreed to discontinue such policies.

One insurance company (the Pearl Assurance Co.) have announced that on all motor insurance policies taken out or renewed after 1 July 1989 they will not be liable for any claims where the driver was guilty of a drink-drive offence. The wording of the endorsement is, 'We will not be liable to make any claim under this policy if at the time of the accident . . . any motor vehicle insured by the policy is being driven . . . by a person (i) after consuming so much alcohol that the proportion of it in his breath, blood or urine exceeds the limit prescribed by Regulations made by the Secretary of State or (ii) who is unfit to drive through drink or drugs or (iii) who without reasonable excuse fails to provide a specimen . . .'. Policy holders when claiming will be required to state whether the police have breathalysed the driver after the accident and whether they are intending to proceed against the driver as a consequence. If the answer to these questions is positive, insurance cover will be suspended in respect of the accident. The insurance company will not pay for repair of the vehicle and while it will deal with claims for injury and damage to third parties it will take steps to recover any sums paid from the convicted driver. If the driver is found not guilty or the prosecution is withdrawn the claim will be dealt with as normal.

The company believe that their new policy will reduce their claims experience and enable then to reduce premiums. Drivers with an insurance policy of this type have extra reason not to drink and drive. The legal implications of this sort of policy have been reviewed.[31] This new approach to motor insurance is extremely interesting and may be a major contribution to reducing the problem of drink-driving in this country.

## ▶ Characteristics of drink drivers

Over the years, an epidemiological pattern (prevalence at a particular time) has emerged regarding drinking drivers. The incidence is greatest between the hours of 10.00 pm and 3.00 am, being concentrated on Friday and Saturday nights. The myth that Christmas is a peak time is clearly not true. Drink-driving is an all-year-round problem particularly at weekends, with the greatest incidence during the summer.

The characteristics and behaviour of drinking drivers have only recently emerged from new sources of data from the Driver and Vehicle and Licensing Centre, the Nottinghamshire Accident Study and roadside surveys in Sussex and Warwickshire.

### The Driver and Vehicle Licensing Centre

The DVLC driving licence records[32] of drink-driving offences now include details of drivers with blood alcohol levels above 150mg/100ml (65μg/100ml Breath Alcohol Concentration) and include driver details such as age, sex, previous convictions, licence status, and so on.

For the year 1984 the greatest incidence of drink-driving offences was in the 20–29 age group which accounted for two-fifths of offenders but only one quarter of licence holders. The 30–50 age group account for two-fifths of offenders and two fifths of all licence holders. Only 5 per cent of offenders were women although 41 per cent of licence holders are women.[33] Whilst the mean alcohol level in those convicted was about 1.9 times the legal limit, the level steadily increased with age up to age 60 after which it fell back.

There appears to be a relationship between drink-driving offences and other motoring offences. Motorists who have been convicted of a drink-driving offence during the past five years were twice as likely to have committed other motoring offences such as careless or reckless driving or accident offences. Those who went on to commit a further drink-driving offence were five times as likely to have committed other motoring offences.[34] This link between drink-driving offences and other offences against the law has been shown by A. B. Clayton to extend also to non-motoring offences[35].

### Nottinghamshire Accident Study

This was carried out over the year 1986–87 and was the first study in Britain to include all accidents and to ascertain driver/rider alcohol levels[36]. This was made possible because of the police force policy of screening wherever possible all drivers involved in accidents. Drinking histories and patterns of drinking, social background and driving experience were explored by interview. Overall, 94 per cent of drivers were found to have Breath Alcohol Concentration below 17.5µg/100ml (half the legal limit), 1 per cent between 17.5 and 35µg/100ml and 5 per cent were above the limit (35µg/100ml).

Men were over-represented in the high breath alcohol category as were the 20–24 age group and drivers/riders from manual occupations (socioeconomic groups IIIM, IV and V. Drivers aged under 20 and over 40 were under-represented in the high breath alcohol category.

The study has also brought to light the high incidence of licence offences. Eleven per cent of those with high breath alcohol either had no valid licence compared to only 1 per cent of those with breath alcohol below 17.5 µg/100ml. Ten per cent of the high breath alcohol group only had a provisional licence compared to 7 per cent of those with the low breath alcohol. Thus unlicensed drivers and to a lesser extent provisional licence holders were over-represented in the high breath alcohol group.

### Roadside Surveys

Roadside surveys have been carried out in both Sussex and Warwickshire[37] during the spring of 1988 when more than 2600 car drivers were asked to participate. Less than 2 per cent of drivers refused to be interviewed and only 1 per cent refused a breath test. Information was sought regarding age, sex, occupation, driving experience, origin and destination of journey, normal drinking habits, understanding and attitude to drinking, and so on. The survey was carried out between 10.00 pm and 3.00 am on Thursday, Friday and Saturday nights over a six-week period.

Once again men were over-represented amongst those who had been drinking, particularly in the 25–39 age range. Overall 95 per cent of drivers had less than half the legal limit, 4 per cent had between half and the limit, and 2 per cent were above the legal limit. Fifty per cent of those who had breath alcohol over the limit could be classified as 'heavy' drinkers. Twenty-seven per cent of these drivers thought they could drink more than five units of alcohol and still be below the legal limit, whereas only 6 per cent of the general driving population held this belief. Forty-four per cent of drivers over the limit felt they could drive safely at the legal limit but only 10 per cent of the sample as a whole thought they could. There was a gross under-reporting of levels of drinking amongst those who had the higher levels of breath alcohol. This study illustrates the need for greater public education and information, particularly in the younger age group.

## ▶ Problem drinker/high risk offenders

Between 2 per cent and 10 per cent of the British population have to a greater or lesser degree experienced a range of problems in respect of their drinking; drinking and driving is simply another of their drink-related problems. Habitual heavy drinkers are particularly likely to have a road traffic accident.[38] A conviction for a drink-driving offence may be the first sign of the problem[39, 40] and could be used to encourage the offender to seek help.

There is a subgroup among drink-drive offenders who have other alcohol-related problems as a result of which they are likely to reoffend when their licences are restored at the end of the period of ban. Under the 1981 Transport Act certain categories of offender (those who are convicted of a drink-drive offence twice within ten years; those with a blood alcohol concentration over 150mg/100ml; and those who refused to provide a breath, blood or urine specimen) may be required to undergo medical examination before their licence is restored. These categories will certainly include a number who have other drink related problems and are therefore at high risk of reoffending.

There are no foolproof criteria which can be used to determine whether any underlying alcohol problem has been resolved and it is misleading to suggest that this question can reliably be answered by medical examination. It should be a matter for the Court to decide whether a driving licence should be restored after a ban imposed for a drink-driving offence. In reaching this decision the Court may consider whether the offender has attended a course for drink-drive offenders, attended an alcohol counselling agency, used self help packs, or taken other steps to resolve an underlying drink problem.

The law should be clarified so that for high risk categories of drink-drive offender the period of suspension is indefinite. Offenders should after a specified time be able to apply to the court for restoration of their licence, and produce evidence that any alcohol-related problem has been resolved.

## ▶ Courses for drink-drive offenders

Various experimental schemes have been established for drink-drive offenders. In Great Britain courses have been run by the Probation Service in Hampshire and by a specialist alcohol agency (Aquarius) in Birmingham.[41] These courses usually include sessions on general alcohol education, the effect of alcohol on driving ability, the law relating to alcohol, driving skills and social skills.

---

*Recommendation No. 28*

It is recommended that special alcohol and driving courses for drink-drive offenders, organised by the Probation Service and other recognised bodies, should be available in all districts. Courts should consider attendance at these courses when determining whether to restore a licence.

---

# ▶ Prevention

In spite of the amount of public educative material available, including the recent drinking and driving national campaigns, there still remains a considerable amount of ignorance regarding the danger of alcohol when associated with driving.[42] There remains also the difficulty of using information to change behaviour – because knowledge does not necessarily influence behaviour: cultural change is required where the separation of drinking and driving is the norm.

The Brewers' Society have produced a booklet[43] and video for young people about drinking and driving. Although helpful, it stresses the need to drink and stay within the legal limit whereas it should be stressing the increased risk of an accident after consuming even small quantities of alcohol. There is much sense in the view that all drivers should be subjected to a 'near zero' legal limit for at least two years after taking their driving test.

The drinks trade has a large part to play in assisting the swing towards the view that drinking and driving do not mix (see Chapter 10). There have been a number of initiatives, for example some public houses promote a special drivers' drinks area which displays low-alcohol and soft drinks, and where exorbitant prices are not charged. However, much still needs to be done by the drinks trade to support the various drink-driving campaigns.

Non-drinking driver schemes should be encouraged, whether by mutual consent and arranged amongst a party of people or private or public transport schemes. Such schemes and options must be available and reasonable in cost.

*Recommendation No. 29*

It is recommended that all public houses should have an attractive, prominently displayed selection of non-alcoholic drinks for drivers, and profit margins on these items should be no higher than margins on alcoholic drinks.

*Recommendation No. 30*

It is recommended that employers who organise office parties or other events where alcoholic drinks are to be served should make arrangements for participants to return home without the need to drive.

## ▶ Driving instruction

Driving instructors have the task of teaching people to drive safely. They should include instruction on the effect of alcohol on driving ability as part of the standard instruction programme. The Highway Code only contains one short section on alcohol and the road user and gives very little practical information. New drivers ought to know how to count their alcohol intake and how many hours it is necessary to wait after drinking before their blood alcohol levels are back to normal. A scheme encouraging driving schools to take on these tasks has already been introduced in the county of Avon and this scheme needs to be extended.

*Recommendation No. 31*

It is recommended that much more information regarding drinking and driving and the legal limits should be included within the Highway Code, and questions regarding this be asked at all driving tests.

References

1.  Transport and Road Research Laboratory, *The facts about drinking and driving* (Crowthorne: Transport and Road Research Laboratory, 1986).
2.  British Medical Association, *The Drinking Driver. Report of the Board of Science and Education* (London: BMA, 1988).
3.  Department of Transport, *Road Accidents of Great Britain 1987. The Casualty Report* (London: HMSO, 1988).
4.  A. Smith and B. Jacobson, *The Nation's Health – A Strategy for the 1990s* (London: King Edward's Hospital Fund, 1988).
5.  Ibid.

6. _Road Accidents of Great Britain_, op. cit.
7. British Medical Association, *The Drinking Driver*, op. cit.
8. Dept. of Transport, Consultation Document on *The Cost of Road Accidents* (London: Department of Transport, 1988).
9. R. F. Borkenstein *et al.*, *The Role of the Drinking Driver in Traffic Accidents, Indiana* (Indiana: Department of Police Administration, 1964).
10. British Medical Association, *The Drinking Driver*, op. cit.
11. Dept. of Transport, *Road Accidents of Great Britain*, op. cit.
12. A. B. Clayton, A. C. Booth and P. E. McCarthy, *A Controlled Study of the Role of Alcohol in Fatal Adult Pedestrian Accidents*, SR332 (Crowthorne: Transport and Road Research Laboratory, 1987).
13. D. C. Stark, *The Risk of Fatal Accidents to Drinking Drivers and Pedestrians*, WP/RS/44 (Crowthorne: Transport and Road Research Laboratory, 1987).
14. Department of the Environment, *Drinking and Driving. Report of the Blennerhassett Committee* (London: HMSO, 1976).
15. L. H. Ross, *Deterring the drinking driver* (Lexington: Lexington Books, 1982).
16. Alcohol Concern, *The Drinking Revolution* (London: Alcohol Concern, 1987).
17. National Opinion Polls (NOP), *Market Research Random Breath Testing: A Survey for the Institute of Alcohol Studies* (London: National Opinion Polls, 1987).
18. L. L. Pendleton, C. Smith and J. L. Roberts, 'Public opinion on alcohol policies', *British Journal of Addiction*, 85(1990) pp. 125–30.
19. R. M. Arthurson, *Blood Alcohol Concentration in Drivers: 0.05 or 0.08* (Australia: Traffic Authority New South Wales Traffic Accident Research Unit PJ11/85, 1985).
20. D. C. Stark, *The Risk of Fatal Accidents*, op. cit.
21. R. M. Arthurson, *Blood Alcohol Concentration in Drivers*, op. cit.
22. British Medical Association, *The Drinking Driver*, op. cit.
23. Anon, *Alliance News*, No. 3696, November 1985.
24. Anon, *The Triple A Review*, vol. 2. (1985) p. 20.
25. Ibid.
26. Ibid.
27. Department of Transport/Home Office, *Road Traffic Law Review Report* (The North Report) (London: HMSO, 1988).
28. B. E. Sabey, J. T. Everest and E. Forsyth, *Roadside Surveys of Drinking and Driving*, TRRL Research Report RR 175 (Crowthorne: TRRL, 1988).
29. Department of Transport/Home Office, *The North Report*, op. cit.
30. Anon, *The Triple A Review*, vol. 2. (1985) p. 20.

31. J. Vann, 'Withdrawal of insurance in drink/drive cases', *Solicitors Journal*, 133(1989) pp. 1464–6.

32. J. Broughton, *Analysis of Motoring Offence Details from DLVC Driving Licence Records*, TRRL Research Report RR 77 (Crowthorne: TRRL, 1986).

33. DVLC, *Statistics on driving licence holders* (London: HMSO , 1988).

34. J. Broughton, *Analysis of Motoring Offence Details*, op. cit.

35. A. B. Clayton, P. E. McCarthy and J. M. Breen, *The Male Drinking Driver: Characteristics of the Offender and his Offence*, TRRL Report SR 600 (Crowthorne: TRRL, 1980).

36. B. E. Sabey *et al.*, *Roadside Surveys of Drinking and Driving*, op. cit.

37. Department of Transport/Home Office, *The North Report*, op. cit.

38. J. A. Dunbar, S. A. Ogston, A. Ritchie, M. S. Devgun, J. Hagart and B. T. Martin, 'Are Problem Drinkers Dangerous Drivers? An investigation of Arrest for Drinking and Driving, Serum Gamma glutmyl Transpeptidase Activities, Blood Alcohol concentration and Road Traffic Accidents. The Tayside Safe Driving Project', *British Medical Journal*, 290(1985) pp. 827–30.

39. Ibid.

40. J. A. Dunbar, B. T. Martin, M. S. Devgun, J. Hagart and S. A. Ogston, 'Tayside Safe Driving Project. Problem Drinking among Drunk Drivers', *British Medical Journal* 286(1983) pp. 1319–22.

41. Aquarius, *CARS (Court Alcohol and Road Safety Courses* (Birmingham: Aquarius, 1989).

42. B. E. Sabey *et al.*, *Roadside Surveys of Drinking and Driving*, op. cit.

43. The Brewers' Society, *Finding out about Drinking and Driving. A Biology and General Studies Resource Book* (London: Brewers Society, 1984).

# ►8► ► ► ► ► ► ► ► ► ► ► ► ► ► ►

# PROVISION OF ADEQUATE AND EARLY HELP

► The need for services for problem drinkers

The broad diversity of problems related to alcohol use requires an equally broad provision of resources to deal with those problems. A strategy which aims to reduce the amount of alcohol consumed overall will do a great deal to reduce the harms associated with that consumption; the educational and fiscal tactics which such a strategy might employ were addressed in Chapters 4 and 6. There remain a number of people whose habit of alcohol consumption already affects, or threatens to affect, the quality both of their own lives and of the lives of their family and friends. Furthermore, such individuals may put the immediate safety of themselves and others at risk, by drinking while driving, or drinking while working. These people need help to modify their habit. This chapter describes the resources that are available, to identify and help those whose drinking habit has already become, or is threatening to become, a serious problem: the 'high risk' approach.

It has been stated repeatedly that heavy drinkers are at one end of a continuous spectrum of drinking, which runs from non-drinkers to those with very severe problems. In the same way, help at an individual level must have the flexibility that will allow a range of intervention, from support given to the family group, to admission to an alcohol treatment unit, while recognising that for many, minimal intervention may be all that is required.

## ▶ A range of services

This chapter considers the range of care in four sections: support and care from family and friends; help provided by the voluntary sector; the role of the primary health care team and occupational health services; and the place of the specialist services. Variety and flexibility of response require constant liaison between the different sections and co-ordination of all aspects of care. Primary care workers require training and support in their role from specialist services, and all services can expect greater success if they have the support and involvement of the family.

In many districts voluntary services are the major available resource for identifying and helping individuals with drink-related problems. The nuances and emphases in the structure of local services will vary from place to place, but the goal of a co-ordinated, flexible and adequate response should remain the same, bearing in mind the principle that, 'Sound planning should result in a little treatment for many and a lot of treatment for a few'.[1]

The process of developing a local strategy for action will be discussed further in Chapter 9.

## ▶ Self help and family support

Inappropriate alcohol use by any member of the family can have serious effects on family life. The associations with severe forms of that harm, such as child abuse or overt violence, have been well rehearsed and graphically illustrated. The grey area between this black picture of violence and the white purity of domestic bliss (in which alcohol may well play a subtle role) contains an amount of stress and disharmony at which one may only conjecture. These issues have been discussed in Chapter 3.

Excessive drinking can, however, be addressed and modified without recourse to outside agencies. The harm that is done to children of a heavily drinking parent, for example, can be very much reduced by the ability of the non-drinking parent to cope with the problem.[2] Spontaneous moderation of drinking habits does occur with time. This was demonstrated in 7735 middle-aged British men who were part of the British Regional Heart Study.[3] The authors observed that over a period of five years, more than 40 per cent of men reduced their drinking, while only 10 per cent increased their intake. Most significantly, the proportion of the sample that were heavy drinkers (over 42 units per week) fell from 10 per cent to 4 per cent of the total (see Figure 8.1). It was noted that a reduction in consumption was most likely to occur in association with the onset of ischaemic (coronary) heart disease; prescription of regular medication; or acquisition of two diagnosed illnesses, irrespective of age. It is difficult to decide whether this change was a result of a changing social environment, or merely a consequence of getting older.

The incidence of heavy drinking and alcohol-related problems has been shown to decrease with age in other longitudinal and cross sectional surveys.[4,5] Alcohol consumption across the United Kingdom did not appear to be falling during the five-year follow-up period of the British Regional Heart Study.[6]

FIGURE 8.1    *Changes in alcohol consumption with ageing*

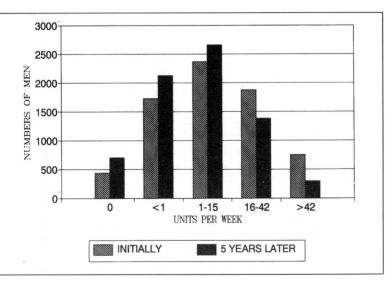

SOURCE    G. Wannamethee and A. Shaper, 'Changes in drinking habits in middle aged British men', *Journal of the Royal College of General Practitioners*, 38(1988).

There has been little examination of what factors influence moderation of drinking habit, other than medical intervention. G. Wannamethee and A. Shaper observed an association with initial heavy drinking, lower social class and intercurrent illness.[7] In 1979, a community survey detected a small number of people who were classed as having had an alcohol problem in the past. A substantial proportion of them had moderated their drinking habits without recourse to medical help; such moderation was associated with significant life events, such as marriage or a change of job. A number of people had received medical help; they were now more likely to be teetotal than the other group, and tended to have had a more chronic problem.[8]

A more recent and much larger survey in the United States involved 774 abstainers, identified in a survey of 5320 individuals. Of the 328 who were current abstainers (as opposed to lifelong abstainers), 41 per cent claimed to have stopped drinking for health reasons, and 20 per cent believed that they had had, or continued to have, a problem with alcohol. Interestingly, the proportion of ex-moderate or heavy drinkers among those who were current abstainers was similar to the distribution of habit amongst current drinkers.[9]

Many individuals who are moderate or heavy drinkers do reduce their consumption, either spontaneously or through a significant change in their social circumstance or state of health. Family and friends can support, encourage or initiate such changes. Awareness of the dangers of alcohol consumption at an individual level is important to this process; the issue of health promotion and public education which promotes that understanding was addressed in Chapter 4.

This process of self-governed remission of excessive consumption is a subject worthy of further research. All who are in a position to lend support or give advice to those families affected by the heavy drinking of one of their members should be encouraged by the knowledge that a high proportion of heavy drinkers will at some stage return to safer drinking patterns.

## ▶ Alcohol and voluntary organisations

The involvement of voluntary organisations with alcohol problems has a very long history. Many of the early ones originated in the temperance movement, but in recent years these have largely been superseded by other modern organisations, using newer concepts of the problem, and different methods.

There is a wide range of voluntary organisations who do work potentially relevant to alcohol problems and it is important to have adequate knowledge of the types of organisation and the particular roles that they fulfil. The term 'voluntary' has become an obstacle to understanding, as it is used with varying meanings. The term is sometimes used to mean agencies which are in the non-statutory sector and non-profit-making, sometimes to mean agencies which use volunteers (that is, non-paid workers), and sometimes with an amalgam of both meanings. Some organisations in the voluntary sector use volunteers, but others do not. The term voluntary is best used to describe organisations working in the non-statutory, non-profit-making sector.

For the purposes of this study the voluntary organisations can usefully be considered in three groups: Alcoholics Anonymous and related organisations; the specialist alcohol agencies; and the relevant non-alcohol specialist agencies.

## ▶ Alcoholics Anonymous

Alcoholics Anonymous (AA) is a famous international organisation which is now reputed to have upwards of a million members. It has a wealth of experience and is potentially a valuable part of local service provision. Alcoholics Anonymous should be encouraged to play their full role alongside other services.

Alcoholics Anonymous works through 'meetings' for members. Sometimes open meetings are also held at which non-members are welcome. The basic principles of the work AA does are described in 'twelve steps', which follow a progression from admitting the power that alcohol has gained, to recognising a 'spiritual awakening' and a determination to carry the message to other 'alcoholics' (see Table 8.1). The language of the twelve steps, and the short, formal prayer which ends each meeting suggest parallels with religion, but the organisation does not require or instil any religious belief.

TABLE 8.1    *The twelve steps of Alcoholics Anonymous*

---

1.  We admitted we were powerless over alcohol – that our lives had become unmanageable.
2.  Came to believe that a power greater than ourselves could restore us to sanity.
3.  Made a decision to turn our will and our lives over to the care of God as we understood Him.
4.  Made a searching and fearless moral inventory of ourselves.
5.  Admitted to God, to ourselves and to another human being the exact nature of our wrongs.
6.  Were entirely ready to have God remove all these defects of character.
7.  Humbly asked Him to remove our shortcomings.
8.  Made a list of all persons we had harmed and became willing to make amends to them all.
9.  Made direct amends to such people wherever possible, except when to do so would injure them or others.
10. Continued to take personal inventory and when we were wrong promptly admitted it.
11. Sought through prayer and meditation to improve our conscious contact with God as we understood Him, praying only for knowledge of His will for us and the power to carry that out.
12. Having had a spiritual awakening as the result of these steps, we tried to carry this message to alcoholics, and to practice these principles in all our affairs.

---

Aside from the coherent strategy of the twelve steps, Alcoholics Anonymous presents an opportunity to make new acquaintances, join a new social group, and regain a sense of personal worth. This approach is very helpful for many but is not appropriate for everyone. Its aim is abstinence rather than moderation. Groups will vary in their social class make up and their emphasis on spirituality.

It is important that professionals working in the field should use Alcoholics Anonymous as an ally on appropriate occasions. Similarly, good liaison will ensure that Alcoholics Anonymous is aware of the various local professional services and can recommend that their help be employed when necessary.

The nature of the organisation of Alcoholics Anonymous is very important to its functions. It is a 'fellowship of recovering alcoholics' and functions entirely by the voluntary efforts of its members. As such, it is an organisation of volunteers, rather than a voluntary sector agency. It does not seek or accept statutory funding and its activities are difficult to plan for in a local service provision plan. Alcoholics Anonymous will usually participate readily in meetings concerned with alcohol problems, but will typically send an 'observer', rather than a person with managerial responsibilities. The orgainisation is very widespread and larger cities will have a number of functional AA groups, which can usually be found in the telephone directory. They are also likely to hold regular visiting meetings in local alcohol treatment units and in prisons.

Al-Anon is an organisation that is independent of, but allied to Alcoholics Anonymous. Following similar principles, it is a self-help group for the families of alcoholics, most commonly wives or girlfriends. Al-Anon groups can provide valuable support in many instances.

Al-Ateen is another independent organisation, working along similar lines, which helps the teenage children of an alcoholic. It is not yet common in Europe, being more widespread in North America.

## ▶ Specialist alcohol voluntary agencies

There are a large number of voluntary sector agencies specialising in alcohol work. All such agencies are likely to be known to Alcohol Concern, the national agency on alcohol misuse, which publishes a directory of alcohol services in England and Wales.[10]; in Scotland the comparable body is the Scottish Council on Alcohol.

The voluntary sector specialist alcohol agencies vary widely in their organisation and methods of working, but variations on the 'local council on alcohol' type of service are to be found in many areas. A local council on alcohol typically consists of a group of concerned and influential people. This council then employs a staff team which usually consists of a director, one or more counsellors and a secretary. In some cases, the employed staff recruit, train and manage a team of volunteers. Local councils on alcohol often operate under the name of 'Alcohol Advisory Service' or a similar title.

These services commonly cover three broad areas: counselling and information for problem drinkers and their families; public education and primary prevention work; and training work for statutory authority staff in dealing with alcohol problems. Staff of some local councils may also develop special expertise in areas such as workplace alcohol policies campaigning, or young people's drinking.

A number of other types of service are provided by voluntary sector agencies. Residential provision includes night shelters, residential care, hostels and housing. Some are provided by specialist alcohol agencies such as Turning Point or Aquarius and others by more general housing agencies such as Stonham. Detoxification or drying out facilities linked to longer-term help are typically provided by local agencies specialising in this work (for example, St Dismas in Southampton or Trinity Centre in Birmingham). The paid staff of voluntary-sector specialist alcohol agencies commonly have a professional background in social work, nursing, counselling or some other caring profession. Alcohol Concern has set up a Volunteer Alcohol Counsellor Training Scheme (VACTS) to set standards and accredit local training schemes for volunteers.

The voluntary sector specialist alcohol agencies are usually funded by a mixture of grants from local authorities, grants from health authorities and charitable donations. The Department of Health provides very limited funds to start new services in areas where they are lacking, through a scheme administered by Alcohol Concern (Section 64 funding).

## ▶ Relevant non-alcohol-specialist agencies

The work of many voluntary sector agencies is relevant to alcohol problems without their specialising in this area. The contribution of the Salvation Army hostels is well known, and many other organisations make major contributions around the country. Their staff need adequate training and proper support in order to deal with alcohol-related issues which they will encounter in their work.

Some general counselling agencies have considerable potential for contributing to prevention and resolution of alcohol-related problems. One such agency is Relate, formerly known as the Marriage Guidance Council. This is increasingly playing a preventive as well as a rescue role, through involvement with local youth organisations, prisons, pre-marital advice, and groups for pregnant women. In some areas, Relate counsellors already work with social workers and ˙primary health care teams. Counsellors are likely to encounter many clients whose drinking patterns are a contributory factor in their problems. They need to be able to recognise the signs of alcohol-related problems, have the confidence to ask about drinking habits and appreciate how best to address those problems, and to decide whether to involve professional help. Relate counsellors could make a significant contribution to the containment of alcohol-related problems by ensuring that the counselling process gave due weight to them.

The Samaritans are another organisation who are likely to encounter many clients with alcohol-related problems in the course of their work. The organisation was established in 1953 with the aim of helping, in particular, people who were in despair to the point of suicide. Alcohol is frequently part of the descent into such despair and often it is the presenting problem. Training for Samaritan volunteers is organised at a local level, but follows national guidelines. All volunteers receive induction training prior to service and subsequently continue to have in-service training. Local branches have a nominated trainer, who would doubtless be willing to discuss the training programme as it relates to alcohol.

## ▶ Alcohol problems and primary care

Primary care is provided by a wide range of disciplines which include general practitioners, health visitors, community nurses, social workers, and community psychiatric nurses. These professionals have a particular part to play in both the detection and curtailment of high risk drinking. It is a legitimate part of their role for them to enquire about alcohol consumption of individuals who come to them, and to intervene (or ask others to intervene) should action be required.

Simple measures taken by primary care workers can be of lasting benefit, as has been demonstrated in a general practice setting. In one study, 909 patients were identified as excessive drinkers and were randomised into 'control' and 'treatment' groups. The 'treatment' patients were given specific counselling by a trained general practitioner, and at least one follow-up appointment was made. After one year, 71 per cent of 'control' women and 75 per cent of 'control' men continued to drink excessively, compared with 52 per cent of 'treatment' women and 56 per cent of 'treatment' men.[11]

In order to achieve success, however, it is necessary first to identify those who are drinking excessively. Heavy drinkers are known to consult their general practitioners more frequently than do light drinkers.[12] Nevertheless, a substantial number of such drinkers may pass unrecognised. In 1986 a paper described the general practitioner assessment of 2081 patients.[13] Only 28 per cent of high-risk drinkers among that sample, and 45 per cent of moderate to heavy drinkers, were identified. In this study, only 54 per cent of those GPs who were invited to take part accepted the invitation, a degree of selection which might be expected to show a higher detection rate than that which exists in reality. In another study, a structured questionnaire was used to assess whether patients presenting to their general practitioner had come because of a 'drug problem' (tobacco, alcohol, caffeine or other).[14] In those patients who did not undergo this formal procedure prior to clinical interview, the GP remained unaware of any problem in 40 per cent of cases. Conversely, exposure to the formal enquiry was a clear encouragement to patients to discuss the relevant substance during the clinical interview. The authors suggested that a brief assessment of lifestyle is possible in any practice setting, and is of significant value.

The Royal College of Physicians recommended that, 'Every person seen in general practice or in hospital should be asked about his or her alcohol intake as a matter of routine, along with questions about smoking and medication, and the answers recorded'.[15] Brief recommendations as to how this should be done are made in the recently issued booklet *Drinking Problems*.[16] The Royal College of General Practitioners discuss the process of such assessment in greater detail.[17] The Faculty of Public Health Medicine supports these recommendations.

Such assessment, however, requires training of all primary care workers so that they are aware of the need to make such enquiry, and confident of their ability to deal with the issues that such enquiry raises. The West Midlands Region, for example, has provided a Regional Alcohol Training Scheme (RATS) with three- and four-day courses and an aim to train 10 per cent of the 'first contact' staff in the region.[18] The English Nursing Board runs specialist courses relating specifically to alcohol problems.

It is particularly important to identify those whose drinking habits place them at slightly elevated risk. The Royal College of General Practitioners discusses this group in terms of low and high vulnerability.[19] Alcohol consumption is a dynamic habit, and timely advice may prevent any deterioration. Furthermore, as has been discussed, a general reduction in consumption at this level of drinking will result in a significant fall in overall alcohol-related illness.

More than 90 per cent of patients on a GP's list are expected to present to the practice at least once in a five-year period. A systematic programme of opportunistic screening has been shown to have a high uptake rate, and would be a valuable tool in assessing and monitoring habits of alcohol consumption. A programme has been described, using nurses in a practice facilitator role, which is a cost-effective and successful method of preventive screening in a primary care setting.[20]

It is important that all primary care staff work as an integrated team, and that they regard the voluntary agencies and secondary care services as allies, to be used and consulted whenever appropriate. Recommendations have been made that will encourage and support this process.

---

*Recommendation No. 32*

It is recommended that regular training opportunities should be provided for primary care workers to develop their knowledge of alcohol-related problems and their skills for intervention in such problems.

> **Recommendation No. 33**
>
> It is recommended that all Family Health Service Authorities and District Health Authorities should encourage and support programmes of screening and health education, in a primary health care setting, for those populations for which they are responsible.

## ▶ Alcohol and occupational health

Many problem drinkers are employed. The costs of excessive drinking are high both to individual drinkers and to their employers.[21, 22] A joint report produced by the Department of Employment, the Health and Safety Executive, and the Department of Health and Social Security called for unions and employers to develop policies which would encourage problem drinkers to come forward for help without threat to their prospects or their livelihood.[23] Such policies are widespread in the United States and elsewhere, and are increasingly common in Great Britain. The nature of such policies will be discussed in Chapter 9.

The detection and treatment of problem drinking at work is an important part of overall local action, especially in areas with large single employers. The principles of screening by occupational health staff, of the training of these staff, and of good liaison between occupational health services and other organisations involved in the problems of excessive drinking, apply in an occupational setting as much as in any other.

Links between health professionals and industry in their locality may be made through several agencies, in particular the area office of the Health and Safety Executive, the Employment Medical Advisory Service, Environmental Health Departments, trade unions, Chambers of Trade, and Chambers of Commerce.

## ▶ Alcohol and general hospitals

Heavy drinkers have an increased risk of suffering from accidents and from a wide range of non-psychiatric illnesses (see Chapter 2). These conditions frequently require attendance at a general hospital as an accident and emergency patient, an out-patient or an in-patient. Each of these contacts represents an opportunity for any underlying drinking problem to be recognised, and for simple intervention. It is sad that this opportunity is so rarely taken.

Taking a simple drinking history will identify patients with risky drinking patterns, yet most patients do not have such a history taken. Attendance at hospital prompts many patients to consider the healthiness or otherwise of their lifestyle and simply raising the issue of drinking and its effect on health may be sufficient to encourage a reduction in alcohol consumption.[24] All hospital doctors, regardless of their speciality, ought to be aware that risky drinking may contribute to the ill-health of their patients. They should be prepared to discuss drinking with their patients, to recognise drinking problems where they exist, and to offer appropriate interventions.

Data on the role of alcohol in admissions to acute, non-psychiatric hospitals is hard to come by. Routine statistics may be misleading and though many in-patients have some characteristics of problem drinkers (see Chapter 2) very few will be recorded as having an alcohol-related problem. Surveys of in-patients' drinking habits do not assess the role of alcohol in each subject's admission.[25] A significant minority of admissions to non-psychiatric hospitals may be for a primary diagnosis of alcohol abuse but have no secondary diagnoses warranting hospital care.[26] Such admissions may incur considerable cost.

## ▶ Care of problem drinkers by psychiatric services

Psychiatric services for problem drinkers include out-patient services, day-patient services and in-patient services. Psychiatrists have played a prominent part in the development of services for those with alcohol-related problems and different units offer a wide range of interventions and therapeutic approaches.

In the 1950s a number of Alcohol Treatment Units (ATUs) were established in the National Health Service. These were intended both to offer services for people with drinking problems and to be centres for education, training and research in the treatment of such patients.[27] However, general psychiatric services continued to see many patients with alcohol-related problems.

A growing number of authorities came to question the appropriateness of the ATUs, which were criticised for offering expensive institutional treatment for a highly selective group of patients and which achieved no better results than much cheaper alternative services.[28, 29] A sentence from the Royal College of Physicians' report summarises the concerns: 'At present, a disproportionate amount of time and money is devoted to the medical treatment of a small proportion of individuals with severe alcohol-related problems, and the generally poor results have led people to question the value of medical treatment'.[30]

The treatment of alcohol abuse is the subject of much debate. The conviction that in patient regimens of counselling and other therapies are the most appropriate forms of treatment is open to question. In 1979, R. E. Kendell said, 'whenever two forms of treatment have been compared . . . the simpler regimen has almost invariably proved to be as effective as the longer or more intensive one'.[31] Subsequent trials have conformed to this pattern.[32, 33, 34] G. Edwards concluded that there is no single answer to the question of what treatment works for highly dependent patients but that a 'flexible and consumer orientated approach that seeks to mobilise natural processes of healing' is required.[35]

There is a body of opinion that the majority of alcohol problems are most effectively managed in the community[36, 37, 38, 39] by multidisciplinary Community Alcohol Teams (CATs). It was suggested that the psychiatrist and psychiatric nurses should become members of a team of professionals who assist primary care agents in dealing with problem drinkers and alcohol dependent individuals.[40] A population of 200,000–300,000 would adequately be served by a team led by one physician or psychiatrist, with access to 4–6 hospital beds which would provide only short-stay, emergency treatment for alcohol abuse.[41] In this plan of services for those with alcohol-related problems the hospital-based psychiatric services are fully integrated with community services and the combined services offer a comprehensive pattern of care.

Such a change in the approach to alcohol-related problems is similar to the change which has occurred in the approach to many psychiatric conditions, with the focus being switched from hospital to community-based care. This is to be supported, although it must be recognised that for a minority, longer-term residential care may still be appropriate.

## ▶ A planned and integrated service

The development of service provision for alcohol-related problems has been piecemeal. A national review by Alcohol Concern found services generally to be patchy, uncoordinated and inadequate in scale.[42]

A comprehensive service would provide a range of different services for clients or patients. The components of such a service are shown in Table 8.2. Every district should have client services and prevention services. They should also have access to a range of services which may be shared between several adjacent districts rather than provided in every district. These services are: workplace services, alcohol training, more intensive client services, Court work, residential services, services for ethnic minorities, services for the homeless, and drying-out facilities.

These services could be provided entirely by statutory agencies such as the National Health Service, local authorities and the Probation Service, or entirely by the voluntary sector. The best arrangement, however, is likely to be an integrated service with some elements provided by the statutory sector and others by the voluntary sector agencies. This arrangement has the advantage of setting the voluntary sector agencies in their proper role of service agencies contracted to provide components of an overall service rather than as groups of enthusiasts worthy of support for unspecified good works.

The cost of providing a comprehensive service has been estimated to be about £190,000 for a district with a population of 250,000.[43] Central government funding would do much to promote development of proper services.

---

*Recommendation No. 34*

It is recommended that each district and region should produce costed plans for the development of a comprehensive range of services for the prevention and management of alcohol-related problems and that the Government should provide funding to enable those plans to be implemented.

---

149

TABLE 8.2   *Components of a comprehensive alcohol service*

---

*Services located in every district (population 250,000)*

1.   *Client services*
     Counselling and advice for problem drinkers and their families.

2.   *Prevention services*
     Preventive work at a local level and public alcohol education.

*Services shared between 3 or 4 adjacent districts (poulation 1 million)*

3.   *Intensive client services*
     Individual and group counselling, day centre facilities and so on, to meet
     a wide range of client needs and particularly to cater for clients with
     more extensive needs. (Combined in some cases with residential
     provision, a special women's service, and so on).

4.   *Residential services*
     Residential care for problem drinkers who need this environment, or who
     are homeless.

5.   *Ethnic minority services*
     Work concerned with alcohol problems in ethnic minority communities
     and the need to develop services, staff training, alcohol educational
     materials and community liaison appropriately.

6.   *Court alcohol services*
     Assistance to the Courts and other legal processes in dealing effectively
     with alcohol-related offending.

7.   *Training*
     Training for all primary level staff of the health authorities and local
     authorities and other agencies, whose work brings them into contact
     with the public, or who are managers of such staff.

8.   *Workplace services*
     The facilitation of workplace alcohol policy development, including
     arrangements for management training, employee education and client
     referral.

---

References

1. Craig M. Sanchez, 'The Hitch Hiker's Guide to Alcohol Treatment', *British Journal of Addiction*, 81(1986) pp. 597–600.
2. C. Wilson and J. Orford, 'Children of alcoholics', *Journal of Studies in Alcohol*, 39(1978) pp. 121–42.
3. G. Wannamethee and A. Shaper, 'Changes in drinking habits in middle aged British men', *Journal of the Royal College of General Practitioners*, 38(1988) pp. 440–2.
4. K. Fillmore, 'Prevalence, incidence, and chronicity of drinking patterns and problems among men as a function of age; a longitudinal and cohort analysis', *British Journal of Addiction*, 82(1987) pp. 77–83.
5. Office of Population Censuses and Surveys (OPCS), *General Household Survey 1984* (London: HMSO, 1985).
6. Office of Health Economics, *Alcohol: Reducing the Harm*, Studies of Current Health Problems No. 70 (London: Office of Health Economics, 1981).
7. G. Wannamethee and A. Shaper, 'Changes in drinking habits', op. cit.
8. W. Saunders and P. Kershaw, 'Spontaneous remission from Alcoholism; a community study', *British Journal of Addiction*, 74(1979) pp. 251–65.
9. E. Goldman and J. Najman, 'Lifetime abstainers, current abstainers, and imbibers – a methodological note', *British Journal of Addiction*, 79(1984) pp. 309–14.
10. Alcohol Concern, *Alcohol Services: A Directory for England and Wales* (London: Alcohol Concern, 1986).
11. P. Wallace, S. Cutler and A. Haines, 'Randomised controlled trial of general practitioner intervention in patients with excessive alcohol consumption', *British Medical Journal*, 297(1988) pp. 663–8.
12. I. C. Buchan, E. G. Buckley, G. L. S. Deacon, R. Irvine and R. Ryan, 'Problem drinkers and their problems', *Journal of Royal College of General Practitioners*, 31(1981) pp. 151–3.
13. A. Reid, G. Webb, D. Hennrikus, P. Fahey and R. Sanson Fisher, 'Detection of patients with high alcohol intake by General Practitioners', *British Medical Journal*, 2(1986) pp. 735–7.
14. H. Skinner, B. Allen, M. McIntosh and W. Palmer, 'Lifestyle assessment; just asking makes a difference', *British Medical Journal*, 290(1985) pp. 214–16.
15. Royal College of Physicians, *A great and growing evil: the medical consequences of alcohol abuse* (London: Tavistock, 1987).

16. Standing Medical Advisory Committee to the Secretaries of State for Health and for Wales, *Drinking Problems: A challenge for every doctor* (London: HMSO, 1989).

17. Royal College of General Practitioners, *Alcohol – a balanced view*. Report from General Practice 24 (London: British Medical Association, 1986).

18. P. Mason, *Managing drink* (Birmingham: Aquarius, 1989).

19. Royal College of General Practitioners, *Alcohol – a balanced view*, op. cit.

20. E. Fullard, G. Fowler and Gray Muir, 'Promoting prevention in primary care; controlled trial of low technology, low cost approach', *British Medical Journal*, 294(1987) pp. 1080–2.

21. S. Holtermann and A. Burchell, *The costs of alcohol abuse* (London: DHSS, 1981).

22. A. Maynard, *Alcohol use: costs and benefits* (London: Alcohol Concern, 1985).

23. D of E, HSE and DHSS, *The problem drinker at work: guidance on joint management and trade union cooperation to assist the problem drinker* (London: HMSO, 1981).

24. P. Wallace *et al.*, 'Randomised controlled trial of GP intervention', op. cit.

25. A. Scheffler, A. Fawcett, J. Pushkin, K. Zahir and M. Morgan, 'Alcohol-related problems amongst selected hospital patients and the cost incurred in their care', *British Journal of Addiction*, 82(1987) pp. 275–83.

26. A. Ogborne and A. Manuella, 'The use of hospital beds for the treatment of excessive drinkers without serious medical complications', *British Journal of Addiction*, 82(1987) pp. 193–6.

27. M. Glatt, *Alcoholism* (London: Hodder and Stoughton, 1982).

28. H. Annis, 'Is Alcoholism Treatment Effective?', *Science*, 236(1982) pp. 20–22.

29. Alcohol Concern, *Alcohol Services: The Future* (London: Alcohol Concern, 1987).

30. Royal College of Physicians, *A great and growing evil*, op. cit.

31. R. E. Kendell, 'Alcoholism: a medical or a political problem?', *British Medical Journal*, i(1979) pp. 367–71.

32. J. Orford and G. Edwards, *Alcoholism. A comparison of treatment of advice, with a study of the influence of marriage* (London: Oxford University Press, 1977).

33. J. Shore and L. Kofoed, 'Community Intervention in the treatment of alcoholism', *Alcoholism: Clinical and Experimental Research*, 8(1984) pp. 151–9.

34. J. Chick, G. Lloyd and E. Crombie, 'Counselling problem drinkers in medical wards', *British Medical Journal*, 290(1985) pp. 965–7.

35.  G. Edwards, 'Which treatment works for drinking problems?', *British Medical Journal*, 296(1988) pp. 4–5.
36.  Office of Health Economics, *Alcohol: Reducing the Harm*, op. cit.
37.  Royal College of Physicians, *A great and growing evil*, op. cit.
38.  D. Raistrick, 'Substance problems: the future of specialist services', *British Journal of Addiction*, 83(1988) pp. 349–50.
39.  World Health Organisation, *Problems related to alcohol consumption*, WHO Technical Report, Series 650 (Geneva: WHO, 1980).
40.  Royal College of Psychiatrists, *Alcohol – our favourite drug* (London: Tavistock, 1986).
41.  Royal College of Physicians, *A great and growing evil*, op. cit.
42.  Alcohol Concern, *Alcohol Services: The Future*.
43.  Alcohol Concern, *A strategy to deal with Alcohol Problems at a Local Level* (London: Alcohol Concern, 1988).

OTHER SOURCES

P. Tether and D. Robinson, *Preventing alcohol problems: a guide to local action* (London: Tavistock, 1986).
G, Edwards, *The treatment of drinking problems. A guide for the helping professions* (London: Blackwell Scientific Publications, 1987).

# ▶9▶ ▶ ▶ ▶ ▶ ▶ ▶ ▶ ▶ ▶ ▶ ▶ ▶ ▶

# LOCAL ACTION TO LIMIT HARM

## ▶ Levels of prevention

A good deal can be done at a local level to prevent alcohol-related problems and to limit the harm incurred. Prevention work may be classified as primary, secondary or tertiary. In the context of alcohol-related harm, primary prevention is focused on people who have not yet experienced such harm, usually children or young adults. Secondary prevention is concerned with the drinking population, many of whom will have experienced transient or reversible harm, which may range from an inconvenient hangover to a driving disqualification. Tertiary prevention focuses on identified problem drinkers who have suffered appreciable harm and for whom the aim is to limit further damage.

While it is useful to categorise preventive action in this way the distinctions will not always be clear and the merits of one category of prevention cannot be weighed against those of another category. The work of some staff will be concentrated in one area of prevention only, but others will span the whole range. The latter may include both specialists and generalists. Thus specialist alcohol agencies are expected to make contributions at all three preventive levels, as are general practitioners and primary health care teams.

Whatever the level of preventive activity it is vital that staff should understand the particular role they are fulfilling and should have a range of skills and methods appropriate to that task. Workers who span several levels of prevention will require a wide understanding and a repertoire of skills and methods.

## ▶ Primary prevention is not enough

Preventing problems from occurring at all may seem preferable to simply limiting the extent of problems which have occurred. However, in the case of alcohol problems this is not practicable. While we work to develop more effective primary prevention there can be no escape from the responsibility for secondary and tertiary activity. Work with small numbers of chronic problem drinkers may seem to be a poor investment of preventive activity, but such individuals can incur considerable further harm and make enormous and costly demands on health and other services. Provision of services for these chronic problem drinkers can thus be cost effective for the community as well as helpful to the individual.

## ▶ Local policy and strategy statements

The list of people and agencies who have a contribution to make to the reduction of alcohol-related harm in the local community is a very long one (see Table 9.1). Working out a local policy and strategy may serve a number of functions. It allows all those who can contribute to meet and exchange ideas, it ensures common ownership of the problem and of the proposed solutions, it prevents wasteful duplication of effort and possible conflicting approaches, and it helps people be clear as to who has taken responsibility for doing which job.[1] The joint strategy produced for Oxford[2] is an example of how different agencies can devise a plan for working together.

Local policy and strategy statements have to take account of local conditions as each district will have different resources and different problems. The difficulty of gaining commitment to a joint approach is illustrated by the many areas in which it has not been achieved. Traditional rivalries between agencies and between departments within agencies, distrust between different professional groups, different methods of working, and over-lapping of boundaries may all complicate the task. The most favourable situations for joint local action is where the local agencies have a history of collaboration and where the local community has a strong sense of identity and coherence.

TABLE 9.1    *People and agencies who could be involved in a local alcohol strategy*

---

*Health authority and family health service staff*
  Public health doctors, general practitioners and the primary care team, Doctors and nurses in general hospitals, psychiatrists and psychiatric nurses, community nurses, health visitors and health education staff

*Local authority staff*
  Social services staff, education department and teachers, recreation and leisure staff, environmental health officers, road safety officers, youth workers

*Police*

*Probation*

*Licensing justices and other magistrates*

*Health and safety at work executive*

*Voluntary sector organisations*
  Specialist alcohol agencies, child-care agencies, agencies for the homeless
  Community organisations
  Neighbourhood groups, churches and religious groups, ethnic community groups

*Trade unions*

*Trade organisations*
  Brewers, licensed victuallers' association

---

One initial obstacle to developing a broad alcohol strategy is the difficulty in altering the common perception that alcohol problems centre on small numbers of 'alcoholics'.[3] The development of a local strategy needs to confront this issue and build up the general understanding that the bulk of alcohol-related harm stems from the drinking habits of large numbers of the general population. The impact of these drinking patterns can then be appreciated in terms of road safety, employment, economics, crime prevention, health and other ramifications. The outcome of the exercise should be that those powerful institutions of the community which often fail to see alcohol-related harm as their concern commit themselves to taking steps to reduce this harm wherever it falls within their remit. If it is to have any impact the scale of activities generated by a local alcohol strategy must be much greater than the small specialist alcohol agencies can ever muster.

The joint departmental circular on alcohol misuse issued in February 1989[4] suggested that a meeting of relevant statutory and voluntary sector agencies should be convened and meet regularly in order to produce and oversee the implementation of a joint strategy. This task would involve collection of data, planning, setting up services and activities, monitoring their effects and reporting back. Although the circular was very general, it could be used to mobilise commitment to a strategy and the necessary action. In some districts there may already be an existing sub-group or forum to which these tasks could be delegated.

*Recommendation No. 35*

It is recommended that local action groups should be set up in every area. These should include the health authority, the local authority, the specialist voluntary organisations, the police, the Probation Service and other interested parties. The task of this group should be to produce an integrated strategy for alcohol-related problems. The strategy should address both prevention of such problems and remedial services for those who already have problems.

*Recommendation No. 36*

It is recommended that the same group should regularly review service provision and preventive activities and monitor the implementation of the strategy.

## ▶ Examples of local action

The rest of this chapter will describe various examples of action taken at a local level. Fuller accounts of these and other examples will be found in two excellent books by P. Tether and D. Robinson[5,6] to which reference can be made.

## ▶ Collection of local data

An essential step in devising a local strategy is the collection of local data. Even when some of these data are not available the exercise of asking is useful since it reminds people of the impact of alcohol on their services. This should include some estimate of the size of the problem. Some items of data which may be available are listed in Table 9.2. Estimates of the numbers involved can also be made by applying national rates for different problems to local populations. Quantitative data of this type should be supplemented by qualitative data such as which issues are seen as priorities by local communities. Data should also be collected on the existing services. Once local data have been collected the information can be used both to implement the planning process and to generate local interest and support for the alcohol strategy.

TABLE 9.2  *Local statistics on alcohol-related problems*

---

*Health authority*
   Deaths attributed to alcohol-related diagnoses
   Admissions to hospital for alcohol-related diagnoses

*Police*
   Convictions and cautions for drunkenness
   Convictions for drink drive offences

*Probation*
   Numbers of probation clients where alcohol is an issue *

*Alcohol agencies*
   Numbers of clients using services

*Coroner*
   Alcohol-related fatal accidents *

*Social services*
   Number of cases where alcohol is an issue *

---

* In many districts this information will not be available but it might be possible to collect it in future.

## ▶ Alcohol education in local schools

The principles of alcohol education in schools were discussed in Chapter 5. There is no reason to expect that teaching children about alcohol will in itself prevent alcohol problems in later life, and where programmes have been evaluated they appear to have had little effect on alcohol use.[7] The hope must be that such education will provide a basis for informed decisions about drinking in later life, taking into account the information and range of choices which are then available. Education about alcohol and other drugs must be integrated into the curriculum.

Local interests in this process can be focused upon ensuring that alcohol education is actually provided in schools and is properly integrated. Local arrangements have to be made to ensure that teachers get any assistance they need in understanding alcohol and its effects. Drug education co-ordinators, and joint posts between local and health authorities or voluntary agencies have demonstrated their usefulness in helping schools and teachers develop effective alcohol education programmes in schools. The excellent materials for alcohol education produced by TACADE (Teachers' Advisory Council on Alcohol and Drugs Education) have been used in many schools.

*Recommendation No. 37*

It is recommended that local education authorities and Boards of Governors should ensure that alcohol issues are explored in their schools and that children have an opportunity to acquire the skills and knowledge that will enable them to make healthy choices about alcohol in later life. The local education authorities should offer teachers appropriate training and support for this work.

## ▶ Local work with young people

Work with young people is another area where there is extensive scope for local initiatives but sensitive planning is needed in order to make it effective. If adults wish their well intended messages to be heard by young people they must be aware of the preoccupations of those young people.[8] The message should be one which can be assimilated within the existing interests of the target group and there needs to be some way of getting it heard through the clamour of commercial and other pressures on young people's attention.

There are good accounts of message targeting and the use of competitions and other media to carry the message. Using sports, musical or popular television personalities is an obvious way to gain attention.

Youth workers need to be aware of alcohol issues and to have the confidence and skills to discuss these issues with their groups. Local arrangements can be made to train youth workers in these areas. They also need to know that if they encounter any alcohol-related difficulties which they cannot handle they can turn to a network of specialist alcohol workers for fast, sympathetic and expert help.

An important resource which has not yet been successfully harnessed in this area is the enthusiasm and energy of young people themselves. Their willingness to work for causes in which they believe is well known and young people are far more likely to identify with and respond to activities led and managed by their peers. Students and other young people have often been the moving forces in local alcohol education activities.

## ▶ Providing alternatives

An interesting development in recent years has been recognition of the importance of alternative courses of action, rather than relying on exhortation. Counselling staff spent time helping problem drinkers to discover that they do have alternatives to drinking and that they do have other ways of responding to their feelings of anger, loneliness, anxiety or whatever.

The 'alcohol-free pub' is a leisure facility with the ambience of a pub except that it does not serve alcoholic drinks. These or other social venues have seen considerable development in recent years and a good deal of experience in their management and the provision of the appropriate music and atmosphere should be available.[9] The main difficulty seems to be in making them economically viable without subsidy or cheap labour. In this respect there may be benefit in linking the 'alcohol-free pub' with a well frequented venue such as a sports centre or skating rink. The increasing availability of alcohol-free beers, lagers, wines (discussed in Chapter 10) adds to the range of products which can be sold in 'alcohol-free pubs'.

There may be more scope in the provision of alternatives than has yet been explored. Many activities such as dancing, listening to pop music, and playing or watching many sports have become strongly associated with heavy drinking so that people find it difficult to enjoy those activities without joining in the drinking. For instance boys who are keen to play rugby and join rugby clubs soon find that if they are to be fully integrated into the team they are expected not only to play well during the match but also to drink heavily afterwards. International class players tend not to be heavy drinkers but at lower levels the two activities are often strongly associated in the subculture. We need to find ways of dissociating these other activities from drinking so that while those who wish to enjoy drinking have the facilities to do so, those who wish to enjoy the activities without drinking are not made to feel uncomfortable.

---

*Recommendation No. 38*

It is recommended that local authorities should review provision of facilities in their areas to ensure that the young have several choices of venue for relaxation, socialisation and enjoyment where they are not under pressure to purchase and consume alcohol.

---

## ▶ Workplace policies

Awareness of the economic costs to employers of alcohol-related harm has been increasing steadily. Many major employers have policies aimed at identifying alcohol-related work problems and providing help for problem-drinker employees. Investment in a workplace alcohol policy can be cost effective for the employer[10] by reducing the costs of employee absenteeism, ill health, poor work, disciplinary proceedings, dismissal and staff turnover, which are all associated with inappropriate and excessive drinking. Frequently a workplace alcohol policy is a component of an 'employee assistance programme'.

Alcohol Concern provides a consultation and training service for setting up and implementing workplace alcohol policies. Many local alcohol advice services are also able to provide firms with help in this area. There are several useful publications, including one covering both alcohol and drugs, produced by the Institute of Personnel Management[11] and another by the Health Education Authority.[12]

Some employers, including a number of health authorities, have adopted workplace alcohol policies for apparently little more than cosmetic effect. They have a policy on paper but little or nothing has happened as a result of it. A policy document can scarcely be worthwhile if it does not result in a significant number of alcohol problems being identified and dealt with. Policies which merely pick up a very few severe drinking problems which appear as disciplinary cases will have little economic or harm-reduction benefit.

A workplace policy must make provision for the following functions:

(a)  awareness raising campaigns;
(b)  alcohol education for the workforce;
(c)  training for managerial staff in recognition of alcohol-related problems;
(d)  monitoring of performance indicators to detect possible problems;
(e)  advice and counselling for employees with alcohol or other personal problems;
(f)  referral arrangementsto specialist help; and
(g)  arrangement for monitoring and reviewing the policy.

A workplace policy should be discussed and negotiated through the relevant staff and management meetings of the organisation so that it is widely known and accepted. There is a fine balance to be struck between being properly sympathetic to employees with alcohol-related problems without undermining the necessary workplace discipline. It should be applied equally to all levels, from shopfloor to boardroom. It should be seen to function largely as a preventive and early intervention measure, and the employees should see it as increasing their job security rather than threatening it. Health authorities have a particular responsibility to set an example by adopting alcohol workplace policies and ensuring that these policies are made to work effectively.

---

*Recommendation No. 39*

It is recommended that all health authorities and local authorities should have written workplace alcohol policies. They should provide the training, managerial backup and resources necessary for the implementation of these policies. Other large employers in the area should be encouraged to develop similar policies for their own workforces.

---

## ▶ Local licensing forums

The role of licensing magistrates has been discussed in Chapter 5. They receive police reports on alcohol-related crime and disorder and maintain close working relationships with the police and with the licensed trade.

A licensing forum is an informal group which serves to widen the range of concerns and interests relating to licensing and which can usefully be considered in discussions of licensing policy. Thus the concerns of medical practitioners, alcohol problem agencies, youth workers and others can be voiced and considered relative to local licensing policy in such a forum.

The Sheffield Licensing Forum has been in existence for several years and meets periodically. Having stimulated interest its geographical scope has gradually extended beyond Sheffield to cover Northern England and the Midlands. It remains to be seen whether the benefit of wider geographical influence compensates for the loss of local focus on one Bench servicing one community. It is true that the Sheffield Forum, having widened its geographical spread, is still operating while other forums which remained local to one community no longer function.

The Home Secretary has recently pointed out to Magistrates the powers which licensing magistrates have to take account of offences such as drink driving associated with particular premises, in the consideration of licensing decisions. For the most part these powers have been little used. The development of the licensing forum idea could contribute considerably to making licensing decisions more responsive to the needs of harm reduction in the locality.

## ▶ Drinkwise campaigns

The nature of and rationale for Drinkwise campaigns were discussed in Chapter 4. The first National Drinkwise Day, on 20 June 1989 consisted of many local campaigns which were co-ordinated with a national campaign run by the Health Education Authority and Alcohol Concern. The initial aims of Drinkwise 1989 are not concerned with prevention or harm reduction, but more modestly and appropriately with individual awareness raising. The messages to be conveyed were decided at a national level and focused on ideas of 'being a better judge of your alcohol consumption' and 'knowing your limits for sensible drinking'.

Successful events require several different agencies such as health authorities, local authorities, police and voluntary sector agencies to pool their resources. They also require someone with tact and vision to co-ordinate the contributions of these various agencies with their very different methods of working. The national campaign can create a fertile environment for local campaigns by stimulating media interest and supplying posters and other campaign materials. A possible drawback of national co-ordination is that it may restrict the ability of local Drinkwise to choose the optimum local time or capitalise on local issues.

It is important that those engaged in local campaigns do not have unrealistic expectations. Public drinking behaviour and attitudes to drinking can only be expected to change gradually. Local preventive activity must try 'to work with the forces of change, not against them'.[13] Since local workers are unlikely to see their efforts rewarded with dramatic change it is doubly important that they should be rewarded with thanks.

*Recommendation No. 40*

It is recommended that health authorities, local authorities, specialist voluntary agencies and other interested parties should co-operate to mount regular campaigns to increase awareness and knowledge of the risks associated with heavy drinking and to promote low-risk drinking patterns. These campaigns should serve to reinforce a programme of continuing community work with the same objectives.

## ▶ Local work with ethnic minorities

Work with ethnic minority communities is necessarily local. In any one district there may be just one homogeneous community or several, with differences of language, religion, cultural habits and attitudes to alcohol. While the proscriptions of their religion against alcohol may endow some communities with a considerable resistance to alcohol problems, no community seems to have immunity. Indeed there is evidence of drinking levels comparable to the indigenous white community in some groups of Asian men,[14] with an expectation that they will experience comparable levels of alcohol-related health and other problems. There must be some risk that drinking problems will multiply in some communities which lack cultural models of moderate drinking but are exposed to all the commercial pressures of advertising.

Organising alcohol education work appropriate to particular communities will be more practicable where there are large homogeneous communities than in districts with several small and different communities. In either case it is necessary to consult widely with the community leaders, community relations representatives and relevant agencies in the statutory and voluntary sectors. There is unlikely to be unanimity on the best approach or even on the nature of the problem but while these differences in perception must be taken into account they must not be allowed to obstruct appropriate action.

In some situations action will best be taken by shaping the services of the existing specialist alcohol agencies so that they meet the needs of an ethnic minority community. In other situations it may be better to train and support workers in existing organisations within an ethnic minority community so as to extend their ability to cater for alcohol-related problems within that community.

*Recommendation No. 41*

It is recommended that all those concerned with primary, secondary or tertiary prevention should review the acceptability and relevance of their activities to the local ethnic minority groups. Where necessary steps should be taken to ensure that these services are available to these groups, either by providing them directly or by supporting existing community groups to provide them.

## ▶ Local working with offenders

It is widely acknowledged that much criminal activity is conducted while in a state of intoxication and that many offenders are heavy drinkers. The nature of this association has been explored in Chapter 3. The proportion of offences in general which are alcohol-related probably lies between 30 and 50 per cent. Consequently, a number of local initiatives have been undertaken to try to deal with the drinking behaviour of offenders as they pass through the criminal justice system.[15]

Alcohol education groups are run for offenders by the Probation Service in most areas, sometimes with the collaboration of a specialist voluntary agency. Typically, alcohol education groups are offered as a component of a Probation Order and if the order is accepted attendance is required as a condition of the order. However in a few areas these groups are offered on a voluntary basis. Alcohol education groups run for a fixed period, commonly six or eight weeks. The groups are intended for offenders who have accepted that their drinking habits are an issue rather than for offenders with chronic drinking problems.

Courses for drink drive offenders have been discussed in Chapter 7.

*Recommendation No. 42*

It is recommended that local magistrates should make much wider use of the option of making attendance at an alcohol education group a condition of probation when sentencing offenders whose offending was alcohol-related.

## ▶ Prison and after-care

Most prisons make some kind of provision for inmates with serious alcohol problems, such as a regular Alcoholics Anonymous meeting run by visiting AA members. However, these activities reach only a small proportion of the inmates who might benefit from modifying their drinking, in terms of their re-offending and their health. On release from confinement and a period of enforced abstinence the majority of prisoners are offered a voluntary after-care facility by the Probation Service. However, only a tiny minority become engaged in any kind of after-care which might help with alcohol-related problems. Schemes to improve the use of appropriate after-care by prisoners who are problem drinkers would contribute considerably to reduction of alcohol-related harm.

*Recommendation No. 43*

It is recommended that after-care schemes which offer help with any underlying alcohol problems should be developed for offenders whose offending was alcohol-related .

## ▶ Alcohol and the homeless

The problem of homelessness is often associated with alcohol-related problems. Being in a state of homelessness must be one of the most severe of the many pressures which may lead someone to adopt high-risk drinking patterns. Provision of suitable and accessible housing must be an important step in the alleviation of alcohol-related problems for people in this unfortunate situation.

There are other local measures for the homeless which can make a useful contribution to harm reduction. In any district there should be some agencies, either statutory or from the voluntary sector, which are providing help for homeless people. This might be in the form of a day centre, a night shelter, or providing access to housing association or hostel accommodation. The focus of their work will be caring and catering for the most basic levels of the hierarchy of human needs.[16] People are unlikely to view alcohol as a relevant issue until their needs for warmth, clothing, shelter, food, affection and some self-respect have been met. At the same time it is important that agencies caring for the homeless should recognise when drinking does become an issue for their clients so that they can be supported and encouraged to take further steps to change their drinking habits. Agencies working with the homeless are dealing with a group who are at high risk of incurring severe, chronic, alcohol-related harm. The agencies need to be supported in this work.

## ▶ Drying-out facilities

The provision of somewhere to sober up and somewhere to stop drinking safely can be seen as contributing to tertiary prevention and harm reduction. This facility would have to operate as part of a system of care so that the drinker had somewhere to go after leaving it. There have been occasional examples of different efforts to provide for this type of need. The Leeds Detoxification Centre, Birmingham Trinity Centre, the Southampton Saint Dismas Alcohol Recovery Unit and the South London Drink Crisis Centre are current examples.

The police make use of such centres to take men who are found drunk and incapable. Although a high proportion of such men leave the centre early the following morning a few will make use of the advice, information and access to further help which is offered. The practicality and economics of this type of provision as a contribution to harm reduction requires further exploration. Systems for providing it where needed should be developed.

Some habitual drinkers need a safe environment in which to stop drinking and go through withdrawal. It is disappointing that apart from the few isolated attempts described earlier no effort had been made systematically to provide facilities in the centres of population where they are needed. Here, as in other areas, the provision of treatment and care also contributes to secondary or tertiary prevention.

## ▶ Meetings to elicit and co-ordinate local action

The usual response to most areas of concern is to call a meeting. Such meetings may vary from an *ad hoc* special meeting brought together to focus on a particular concern to a regular and institutionalised meeting such as that of a joint care planning group or a local council on alcohol. All meetings must have a purpose and it is important to match the type of meeting to its purpose.

Some meetings have achieved a good deal by focusing on a topic area, such as drinking and driving or city centre disorder. Such a meeting can bring together those interests within an area which are most relevant to the topic of concern. A drink driving forum can bring together the police, probation, road safety, RoSPA (Royal Society for the Prevention of Accidents), representatives of the drinks industry, the local authorities, health authorities and specialist voluntary agencies. Such a group can bring their particular contributions to bear on a problem of common concern and co-ordinate their activities for greater effect.

References

1. D. Robinson, 'Alcohol problems (1) Prevention at the local level', *Health Trends*, 19(1987) pp. 19–22.
2. Oxford City Council and Oxfordshire Health Authority, *A balanced Alcohol Strategy for Oxford* (Oxford: Oxford City Council, 1988).
3. D. Robinson, 'Alcohol, education and action: shifting emphases', *Health Education Research*, 1(1986) pp. 325–31.
4. Department of Health/Home Office, *Departmental Circular on Alcohol Misuse*, HN (89) 4; LAC (89) 6; HN (FP) (89) 4 (London: HMSO, 1989).
5. P. Tether and D. Robinson, *Alcohol Problems. A guide to local action* (London: Tavistock, 1986).
6. D. Robinson, P. Tether and J. Teller, *Local action on alcohol problems* (London: Routledge & Kegan Paul, 1989).
7. B. N. Kinder, N. E. Pape and S. Walfish, 'Drug and alcohol education programmes: a review of outcome studies', *International Journal of Addictions*, 15(1980) pp. 1035–54.
8. N. Dorn, 'Youth culture in the U.K: implications for health education', *Institute of Health Education*, 14(1981) pp. 77–82.
9. Alcohol Concern, *Alcohol-free bars* (London: Alcohol Concern, 1988).
10. E. G. Lucas, 'Alcohol in industry', *British Medical Journal*, 294(1987) pp. 460–1.

11. F. Dickensen, *Drink and drugs at work: The consuming problem* (Institute of Personnel Management, 1988).
12. Health Education Authority, *Guidelines for local authorities in the development, implementation and evaluation of an alcohol policy for their staff* (London: Health Education Authority, 1989).
13. S. D. Bacon, 'On the prevention of alcohol problems and alcoholism', *Journal of Studies on Alcohol*, 39(1978) pp. 1125–47.
14. H. M. Mather and D. H. Marjot, 'Alcohol-related admission to a psychiatric hospital: a comparison of Asians and Europeans', *British Journal of Addiction*, 84(1989) pp. 327–9.
15. S. Baldwyn and N. Heather, 'Alcohol education courses for offenders: A survey of British agencies', *Alcohol and Alcoholism*, 22(1987) pp. 79–82.
16. A. H. Maslow, 'Theory of Human Motivation', *Psychological Review*, 50(1943) pp. 370–96.

# THE RESPONSIBILITY OF THE ALCOHOL INDUSTRY

The alcohol industry is large, well established and powerful. In 1986/87, tax revenue from alcoholic drink sales was £6,447m, and in 1987 the industry provided jobs for over 1 million people.[1] The structure of the industry is such that a few firms control the bulk of the market. Eighty per cent of the market share for beer, for example, is divided between just six companies (see Figure 10.1). This allows the industry to take up a consistent position and to lobby the Government with considerable success. It should also afford an opportunity for the negotiation of a common approach towards policies for the marketing and distribution of a product which causes society not only harm but also some benefit. This apparently straightforward national situation is complicated by the internationalisation of the

FIGURE 10.1   *Market share (brewery) UK brewers 1985*

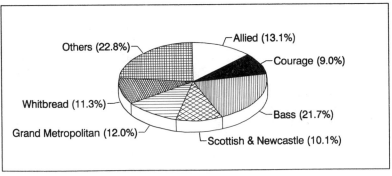

SOURCE   Monopolies and Merger Commission, *Report on Supply of Beers* (London: HMSO, 1989).

industry. The advent of 1992 and an open European market will compound the difficulties of dealing with the industry (whether by negotiation or taxation) at a national level. Furthermore, the increasing corporatism of the large industries, with the industry having interdependent ties with other corporate interests, results in an ownership structure of such complexity that it is difficult to identify a simple set of alcohol industry owners.[2]

## ▶ Social responsibility

It is the paradox of potential for both benefit and harm, discussed elsewhere in this study, that puts alcohol and the alcohol industry in a unique and difficult position, a position very different, for example, from that of cigarette companies. In the case of cigarette smoking, the proper public health position is one of unmitigated opposition to the trade. In the case of alcohol, the proper public health position is to accept that sensible drinking in an appropriate environment is not unhealthy, and that the selling of alcoholic drinks is legitimate and acceptable provided it is done in a socially responsible manner. It must, however, be noted that social responsibility in this activity is of relatively recent origin and still limited in extent.[3]

The alcohol industry must come to this position of compromise from a different point of view. The aim of the industry is inevitably to earn maximum financial return on money invested. To this end it is compelled to achieve as large a volume of sales (at an optimum price) as can be managed. At the same time, the industry must recognise that irresponsible marketing of their product can result in considerable social and physical harm. Such a recognition makes commercial as well as moral sense, since inappropriate behaviour associated with the product would both tarnish its name and invite society to impose its own restraints.

The industry does, in general, accept this dilemma and recognises that it has responsibility for the harmful consequences of the widespread consumption of its products. The two major trade associations (The Brewers' Society and The Wine & Spirit Association) both have committees of social responsibility and meet regularly with those national bodies concerned with the problems related to alcohol consumption. Both are concerned to minimise the damage caused by inappropriate drinking, and have initiated a number of campaigns.[4] The perpetual question is whether the optimum balance between commercial interest, consumer satisfaction, and Public Health has been achieved.

## ▶ Financial support for alcohol agencies

A limited amount of financial support is given by alcohol industry sources for research into alcohol problems (for example, the Alcohol Education and Research Council receives funds from this source), or for agencies working with people with alcohol problems. Many would argue that an industry which makes extensive profits from manufacturing and selling a product ought to contribute generously to the costs of minimising the harm which result from use of that product.

The balance between sales of different drink types (beer, lager, cider, spirits and wines) is changing. The sale of wines has increased considerably over the past decade while that of beer has remained steady. There have also been shifts in the balance between on-licence and off-licence sales. The market share of off-licence sales is also expanding (see Chapter 5). Thus there are pressures of commercial competition within and between elements of the industry which must be taken into account when considering the role of the industry as a whole. That role may be examined by considering its several different aspects.

## ▶ Customer education

When discussing customer education it is necessary to consider the on-licence and off-licence sales separately. It is clear that licensees are in a better position to curb inappropriate drinking behaviour when customers buy it for consumption on the premises than when they buy alcohol to take away for consumption at home or elsewhere.

Those running premises with on-licences have considerable opportunity to control the drinking behaviour of their customers (see the discussion of the drinking environment later on page 181). It is in the licensees' interest to maintain trouble-free premises for the sake of both their custom and their licence.

Brewing companies have considerable influence over the conduct of licensed premises since many licensees are their tenants.

On the other hand, alcohol purchased from off-licence premises will be consumed away from the site of purchase so that the off-licence retailer has little control over the drinking behaviour of his or her customers. Also, the off-licence retailer has less incentive to be responsible since any trouble resulting from consumption of their wares is unlikely to pose any threat either to their licence or to their good name. Furthermore, in 1989, the brewing companies owned only 7 per cent of the 54,000 off-licences so they have little direct influence on how business is conducted in most of these outlets.

The industry has been active in attempting to educate the customers of on-licence premises. In conjunction with the Department of Transport, for example, the Brewers' Society has conducted a series of campaigns, one of which is Wheel-watch. This is an umbrella campaign with two main thrusts, one to promote the sale of low alcohol beverages, the other to promote campaigns to discourage drinking and driving. This campaign is run in conjunction with licensees and the Health Education Authority and is tailored to the needs of local communities. For example, in Norfolk special buses (Boozer Cruisers) were laid on over the Christmas period to allow driving-free revelry, and in Oxford licensees widely advertised and encouraged the use of taxi services by their customers. The Brewers Society also co-operated with the Drinkwise campaign for sensible drinking (see Chapter 4), and has produced quantities of posters and booklets in conjunction with it to explain the meaning of alcohol units and how they should be counted.

It has been difficult to promote such campaigns through off-licence retailers, especially the large supermarkets where alcohol is now commonly sold. The commercial obligations of these retailers are such that promotional material which encourages people to drink (and so to buy) less is unlikely to be welcomed. Nevertheless, the increasing proportion of alcohol consumption that is occurring away from the point of purchase requires that the off-licence retailers acknowledge their responsibility for advising their customers to consume alcohol in sensible quantities and in appropriate situations. The example of Sainsburys stores, who distribute the excellent 'Healthy Drinking' booklet free in their stores, is to be commended.

*Recommendation No. 44*

It is recommended that off-licence retailers should recognise their responsibility to play their part in minimising alcohol-related harm and public disorder. Staff should be trained to exercise responsibility in selling alcohol and that training should become a prerequisite for conferment of a licence.

## ▶ Packaging and labelling

Campaigns of public education can only be a part of an overall strategy to alert people to the pitfalls of inappropriate alcohol consumption. The packaging and labelling of alcoholic drinks is largely irrelevant to the on-licence trade, but may be of great importance to the off-licence trade. The problems of packaging and labelling differ between beer, wine and spirits.

For ten years the specific gravity has been displayed on the bottle or can of alcoholic drink. From 1 July 1989, under an EC (European Community) directive, all packaged drinks must be labelled with their alcohol per centage content by volume. This will be important information for the consumer. Beers may range from 1 per cent to 8 per cent alcohol, wines up to 22 per cent (beyond which they may not be used for human consumption), and spirits from 35 per cent to 45 per cent (but normally sold at 40 per cent).

One of the difficulties of consumption away from the point of purchase is measurement of the amount of drink consumed. Nearly all promotional material, health education campaigns, and recommended safe drinking limits refer to 'units of drink'. For beer these are clearly understood in terms of half pints at a standard strength, and glasses of half pint or pint size are readily recognisable as containing one or two units. Yet standard cans of beer or lager contain approximately two-thirds of a pint and special promotional size cans with 'free 25 per cent extra' or similar complications are not uncommon. This confusion should be ended; containers (cans, bottles, packs, and so on) of beer and similar alcoholic drinks should be labelled with the number of units they contain. Similarly, the chaotic diversity of unit content in different containers and brands should be simplified so that alcoholic drinks were always sold in half 'units', 'units' or simple multiples of 'units'. The law regulates the pack sizes in which washing powder and similar commodities may be sold so that customers are not confused; purchasers of alcohol should be similarly protected.

Bottles of table wine are generally of a standard size and contain approximately seven units. Bottles of fortified wine are more varied in size, but generally contain ten to twelve units. Wine glasses are not all of a standard size, whether for table or fortified wine. To rely entirely on the public perception of 'one standard glass of wine is one unit' in the light of the wide variation in percentage alcohol by volume, and of the variation in glass size, is insufficient. This could be rectified by marking the bottles to indicate the levels of each single unit. Such marking could be done either by etching the glass, or by using appropriate printed labels.

It is difficult to estimate the quantity of spirits poured in the home without the use of a measure or optic. The use of such aids contravenes the conventions of hospitality in our society, which encourage the liberal supply of alcoholic drink to one's guests. Such attitudes should be addressed, and the campaign to do so could be accompanied by a supply of free optics offered through every off-licence retailer. Alternatively, it could be stipulated that every bottle of spirit should incorporate an optic measure which would mete out the drink in single units.

These proposals would involve considerable change in the packaging of alcoholic beverages. Such change is nevertheless required in order that the general public can readily apply the messages of alcohol education campaigns to their own drinking habits. These modifications to the packaging of alcohol would strongly reinforce the message that alcohol consumption needs to be measured and contained whether in a public or a private environment.

*Recommendation No. 45*

It is recommended that alcoholic drink should be packaged and labelled in a manner which makes it easy for the consumer to understand the contents of containers displayed for sale in terms of 'units' or standard drinks. The law should require that alcoholic drinks should be sold in standard quantities of half 'units', 'units' or simple multiples of 'units' and that containers should be prominently marked with the number of units that they contain.

## ▶ Health warnings on containers

One further aspect of labelling is the use of health warnings, for which there is some political support.[5] Such labelling would probably not take the alarming form of those on cigarette packets, but would be similar, for instance, to those on sedative medicines which warn that the substance should not be taken when a person is about to drive or operate moving machinery. This would be of little use in the on-licence trade, but would be a further reinforcement of the sensible drinking campaign as far as the off-licence trade is concerned.

There is an active campaign in the United States for explicit and shocking health warnings to be put on bottles and cans of alcoholic drink. Labels which read, 'Warning: The Surgeon General has determined that the consumption of this product, which contains alcohol, during pregnancy can cause birth defects' have recently been debated in the Senate.[6] The British public is probably not ready to accept labelling of this type.

*Recommendation No. 46*

It is recommended that health labels should be required on containers of alcoholic drinks warning that their consumption will temporally impair ability to drive, work with machinery or do other tasks requiring skill and coordination.

## ▶ Non-alcoholic drinks

The industry has responded well to the growing demand for non-alcoholic or low-alcohol beers and wines (it is highly unlikely that an acceptable non-alcoholic spirit will be developed), and this has had an effect on both the on-licence and off-licence trades. In 1985, for example, there were six brands of non-alcoholic or low-alcohol beers compared with fifty-five brands in 1989. In that time, the share of the beer market taken by low-alcohol beers has grown from virtually zero to 1.5 per cent (Brewers' Society personal communication). The public acceptability of drinking such low- or non-alcoholic wines and beers has been aided both by successful marketing campaigns and by an increasing public awareness of the problems associated with alcohol.

The advantages of alcohol as a social lubricant have been discussed in Chapter 3. The belief that it is the alcohol alone which confers the feelings of well-being and relaxation on the drinker is incorrect. Studies with alcohol-free drinks have demonstrated that the effect of consuming on the drinker is determined to a significant extent by the circumstances and ambience in which drink is consumed independent of the alcohol intake.[7] Non-alcoholic drinks should play an increasingly important role in sensible drinking by the public. Further diversification of the alcohol industry into non-alcohol wine and beer production will allow better reconciliation of their commercial interests with concern for the public health.

## ▶ Advertising

The alcohol industry argues (as does the cigarette industry) that advertising is intended to influence choice of brand (or type) rather than the decision whether or not to drink alcohol at all. Research into this is inconclusive but has been extensively reviewed.[8]

Two studies which took advantage of a complete ban on alcohol advertisements in British Columbia in 1972, and a ban on beer advertisements in Manitoba in 1974[9, 10] illustrate the type of evidence available. Neither study showed an effect on overall consumption but both studies suffered from similar flaws. The population was still exposed to alcohol advertising in neighbouring states; and consumption figures were only monitored for a relatively short time after the bans. The bans might have been expected to affect overall consumption mainly by influencing the annual group of newly legitimised young drinkers and reducing the probability of non-drinkers starting to consume. Any influence on society's overall drinking habits would not be seen until a succession of these groups had reached full adulthood without exposure to the advertisements.

Although brand awareness may be influenced by advertisements in the immediate short term, an effect on overall consumption is more likely to be a subtle, long-term influence. The difficulties of assessing an effect were demonstrated by a survey of print media advertising of alcohol across the United States.[11] No correlation was found between the level of such advertising and the overall per capita consumption, but screen and radio advertising and ethnocultural differences[12] could not be taken into account. There is evidence that choice between drink types (beer, wine, spirits) result in new drink types being added to the types previously consumed, even if brand preference might merely result in one brand being substituted for another.[13] This would certainly explain an effect of brand advertisements on overall consumption.

The British Medical Association advocates a total ban on the advertising of alcoholic drinks. In the legitimate and acceptable trade of alcohol, however, it may be difficult for brands to compete with each other without recourse to advertisement. The Royal College of General Practitioners has expressed opposition to the banning of alcohol advertising on the grounds that the elimination of advertising costs would allow companies to lower their prices.[14] Certainly, the costs to the industry of advertising are not insignificant. A figure has been quoted of £146 million spent in 1985 on press and television advertisement of alcoholic drinks.[15]

The style and content of advertisements are clearly important, and there are standards governing these. The Independent Broadcasting Authority is required by several Broadcasting Acts to lay down a statutory Code of Advertising Standards and Practice, which covers advertisement by television and radio. This code is drawn up after due consultation with industry, consumer groups, medical bodies and other interested parties. Most of the codes are legally binding, although one voluntary agreement is that spirits should not be advertised on television or radio. The Advertising Standards Authority lays down the British Code of Advertising Practice which is not statutory but is a voluntary agreement with industry. This code governs advertising using posters, newspapers and the cinema, and it is very similar to the IBA code.

In general, advertising is not to be directed at the young (the IBA code does not allow the use of actors under twenty-five years of age), is not to associate alcohol with sexual gratification, with driving, or with the control of dangerous machinery, and is not supposed to suggest that consumption of alcohol can potentiate prodigious physical feats. There are some notable omissions, however: these are the failure to ban the association of drinking with other inappropriate activities such as swimming or water sports, and the failure to ban the portrayal of alcohol consumption as an integral part of a desirable lifestyle. It has also been noted that advertisers frequently breach these voluntary codes.[16]

The portrayal of alcohol in the media outside advertisements was discussed in Chapter 4.

> *Recommendation No. 47*
>
> It is recommended that the codes of advertising standards be strengthened and adherence to them closely monitored. If voluntary agreements are not honoured they should be replaced by legally enforceable regulations.

▶ Sports sponsorship

There has been a recommendation that sports sponsorship by alcohol companies should be banned.[17] Already the industry has withdrawn from sponsorship of inappropriate sports such as motor racing. Sports advertising, however, gives access to an important market (sports viewers) for the alcohol industry, such that it is difficult always to make the distinction between what is appropriate and what is not. It seems inappropriate, for example, that a brewery should sponsor a major ocean yacht race when alcohol is such a well-recognised cause of bad seamanship. This year the Football Association have signed an agreement with Tennents' Lager for the sponsorship of the Charity Shield. Such an arrangement seems inappropriate in the light of public concern over drunkenness and disorder amongst football crowds. Sponsorship of this sort is against the interests of public health because it reinforces unhealthy associations of sporting excellence with alcohol consumption.

> *Recommendation No. 48*
>
> It is recommended that sponsorship of sporting events by the alcohol industry should be banned.

## ▶ The drinking environment

One obvious area in which the licensed trade can reduce harm associated with alcohol consumption is by making the drinking environment safer. If someone chooses to drink in a high-risk fashion we may think it better that they did not do so but we must also endeavour to reduce the risk associated with that behaviour. Making the drinking environment safer by careful attention to the social ambience, the surroundings and staff behaviour is one way of reducing risk.

Drinking behaviour and intoxicated conduct are determined by a complex set of unwritten social rules. The choice of beverage consumed is moulded by peer expectations and the social setting. It has been shown that the drinking rate of a group can be speeded up by artificially accelerating the rate of one or two group members.[18]

The surroundings also have a potent effect on behaviour within the drinking environment. Licensees can list the pointers identifying pubs which are unsafe places to drink. These include dirty, peeling wallpaper; damaged seating; a pervasive smell of toilets; uncollected glasses left on tables; noise; large open areas; a clientele which is only of one sex and staff who are scruffy in appearance, frequently intoxicated and indifferent to the behaviour of the patrons. These anecdotal views have been supported by more formal studies from Canada.[19] A useful booklet entitled *Safer Houses* has been produced,[20] aimed at licensees and containing information and checklists designed to help them 'tidy up' the drinking environments they control.

The behaviour of staff also has a very strong influence on the conduct of customers and it has even been claimed that they select regular patrons and determine drinking rates.[21] Staff attitudes and actions will influence how permissive a pub is towards drunkenness and deviant behaviour among patrons.[22]

These conclusions have been culled from studies in many parts of the world and we cannot be sure that what is true in Helsinki or Vancouver applies to a town or city in the United Kingdom. However, enough is known to be sure that there are many actions a licensee can take to reduce the risk that those who drink on their premises will suffer harm or cause harm to others. The licensed trade can work with the local community, in concert with organisations such as the police, the magistracy and environmental health departments to shape the drinking environment and encourage more comfortable and less problematic alcohol use.

### References

1. The Brewers' Society, *Statistical Handbook* (London: Brewing Publications Ltd, 1987).
2. R. McBride and J. Mosher, 'Public Health Implications of the International Alcohol Industry: Issues raised by a World Health Organisation Project', *British Journal of Addiction*, 80(1985) pp. 141–7.
3. R. Weir, 'Obsessed with moderation: the drinks trade and the drink question 1870-1930', *British Journal of Addiction*, 79(1984) pp. 93–107.
4. The Brewers' Society, *Action against Alcohol Abuse. A guide to projects financed by the drinks industry*. Leaflet available from the Brewers' Society, 42 Portman Square, London W1H 0BB.
5. B. Braine, 'Drugs, Alcohol and Tobacco. The Political Dimension', *British Journal of Addiction*, 81(1986) pp. 621–9.
6. S. Blume, 'Warning labels and warning signs: a battle continues across the Atlantic', *British Journal of Addiction*, 82(1987) pp. 5–6.
7. N. K. Mello and J. H. Mendelsen, 'Alcohol and Human Behaviour', in L. L. Iversen, S. D. Iversen and S. H. Snyder (eds) *Handbook of Psycho-pharmacology Drugs of Abuse*, vol. 12., chap. 5., pp. 235–314. (New York and London: Plenum, 1978).
8. R. G. Smart, 'Does alcohol advertising affect overall consumption: a review of empirical studies', *Journal of Studies on Alcohol* 49(1988) pp. 314–23.
9. A. C. Ogborne and R. G. Smart, 'Will restrictions on alcohol advertising reduce alcohol consumption?', *British Journal of Addiction*, 75(1980) pp. 293–6.

10. R. Smart and R. Cutler, 'The alcohol advertising ban in British Columbia. Problems and effects on beverage consumption', *British Journal of Addiction*, 71(1976) pp. 13–21.

11. A. C. Ogborne and R. G. Smart, 'Will restrictions on alcohol advertising reduce alcohol consumption?', op. cit.

12. A. Greeley, W. McCready and G. Theisen, *Ethnic drinking subcultures* (New York: Praeger, 1980).

13. T. Van Iwaarden, 'Advertising, alcohol consumption and policy alternatives', in M. Grant, M. Plant and A. Williams (eds) *Economics and Alcohol: Consumption and Controls* (London: Croom Helm, 1983).

14. Royal College of General Practitioners, *Alcohol – A Balanced View* Report from general practice 24 (London: Royal College of General Practitioners, 1986).

15. B. Braine, 'Drugs, Alcohol and Tobacco', op. cit.

16. L. Pendleton, C. Smith and J. L. Roberts, 'Monitoring alcohol advertisements on television – developing a consensus approach', *Health Education Journal*, 47, pp. 71–3.

17. B. Braine, op. cit.

18. D. A. De Ricco and J. E. Niemann, 'In vivo effects of peer modelling on drinking rate', *Journal of Applied Behavioural Analysis*, 13(1980) pp. 149–52.

19. K. Graham, 'Determinants of Heavy Drinking and Drinking problems: The contributions of the bar environment', in E. Single and T. Storm (eds) *Public drinking and public policy* (Toronto: Addiction Research Foundation, 1985).

20. D. McLean, *Safer Houses: A handbook for licensees on pubs and violence* (Leicester: Leicestershire Alcohol Advice Centre, 1987).

21. E. Single, 'Studies of public drinking, an overview', in E. Single and T. Storm (eds) *Public drinking and public policy*, op. cit.

22. K. Graham, 'Determinants of Heavy Drinking and Drinking Problems', op. cit.

# EDUCATING DOCTORS

▶ Recognising and helping patients with alcohol-related problems

It has been remarked at several points in this study that doctors, both in hospital and in general practice, often fail to recognise the part played by alcohol in their patients' problems. Even when they do recognise alcohol-related problems doctors may be reluctant to intervene.

A study of general practitioners in England[1] investigated some of the reasons for this state of affairs. This showed that although 93 per cent of the general practitioners felt that they had a legitimate role to play in working with drinkers, only 44 per cent felt capable of working with them and only 39 per cent were motivated so to do. A mere 29 per cent of the physicians were satisfied with the way in which they worked with drinkers, and less than one in ten obtained job satisfaction from such work.

▶ Doctors' attitudes to alcohol and alcohol problems

Insufficient knowledge and lack of the skills needed for working with patients with alcohol-related problems are clearly part of the problem but are there more deep seated reasons for the reluctance of doctors to become involved; there are indications that some doctors are confused about their own relationship to alcohol. Alcohol-related problems are the commonest single reason for doctors being reported to the General Medical Council. Alcohol abuse accounted for 48 per cent of cases considered by the Preliminary Proceedings Committee in 1988. Self-help groups have been set up by and for doctors with alcohol-related problems and have reported encouraging results.[2]

Earlier studies in Scotland noted doctors to be 2.7 times as likely as controls in the same social class to be admitted to alcohol treatment units.[3] Doctors used to have much higher cirrhosis death rates than average (SMR (Standardised Mortality Rate) of 350 in 1971) and though this figure has considerably improved (SMR of 120 in 1981)[4] they are still no better than average. The number of doctors with alcohol-related problems has been variously estimated at between 3 and 15 per cent[5] and alcoholism has been called an occupational hazard of the medical profession. If so many doctors are uncertain about control of their own drinking patterns it is not surprising that they can be slow to recognise and help others with alcohol-related problems.

Why do so many doctors drink alcohol unwisely? Doctors with drinking problems are less likely than other people with drinking problems to have a positive family history.[6] Long hours, stress, freedom from supervision and relative financial security may place individuals at risk. These factors apply to doctors and to many other occupational groups. However, medical training at best fails to equip doctors to withstand these pressures and at worst is a factor in the development of alcohol-related problems.

It is to be expected that those recently liberated from school discipline and parental control should experiment with different drinking patterns and sample intoxication. Youthful exuberance exists and no one would wish to deny these pleasures to medical students or other young people. However, in view of the importance of alcohol as a health risk, medical schools should make it plain that they expect their students to develop exemplary drinking patterns. Many doctors who develop drinking problems started drinking heavily at medical school.[7] The stereotype of a medical student as the hard-working, hard-playing, hard-drinking individual immortalised in Richard Gordon's novels is exaggerated but there is still an element of truth.[8] The student arriving at medical school finds most of the opportunities for making friends and meeting socially are also occasions for heavy drinking.

Most heavy-drinking medical students mature to become good doctors with low-risk drinking patterns. However, a sizeable minority come to depend on heavy drinking to relieve stress or to enable them to relax, and they then carry this disability for the rest of their professional life. The greatest problem lies not in the small minority of doctors who drink to excess but in the many doctors who may acquire attitudes to alcohol and alcohol-related disorders that disable them from making a useful contribution to the reduction of alcohol-related harm and from assisting patients with drink-related problems.

## ▶ Educational needs of doctors

Doctors' training should equip them with knowledge, skills and attitudes which will enable them to recognise and help patients who have alcohol-related problems or risky drinking patterns. It should also equip them to play their part in supporting public health measures to reduce alcohol-related harm. The knowledge and skills required are listed in Table 11.1.

Equally important are the attitudes: that alcohol is a substance which if used has to be used with care; that the duty to provide patients with best possible care will require doctors not to drink

TABLE 11.1 *The alcohol knowledge and skills which should be covered in the undergraduate medical course*

KNOWLEDGE
Pharmacological actions of alcohol
Acute toxic effects of alcohol
Organ systems affected by alcohol and alcohol-related diseases
Psychological presentations of alcohol abuse
Social, criminal and employment problems associated with alcohol use
Epidemiology of alcohol consumption and alcohol-related harm
Different types of help available to problem drinkers
Cultural significance of drinking behaviour
Different models of excessive drinking
Public policy options for reducing alcohol-related harm
Alcohol content of different drinks

SKILLS
Take a drinking history
Diagnose the commoner physical diseases associated with alcohol
Simple counselling skills

alcohol if they expect to have to do clinical work soon after; that a doctor's duty is to help patients overcome alcohol-related problems and not to pass judgement on whether or not they are deserving of help. Attitudes will be influenced far more by the prevailing culture and norms than by any formal teaching.

We must look to the education of doctors to find ways of making them more effective in preventing alcohol-related harm and in helping patients with alcohol-related problems. There are three stages in medical education:

1. Undergraduate medical education
2. Higher medical training (postgraduate)
3. Continuing training

## ▶ Undergraduate medical education

Aspects of alcohol appear in many parts of the medical curriculum and are taught in an *ad hoc* fashion by teachers from many disciplines including biochemists, general physicians, general surgeons, paediatricians, hepatologists (liver specialists), pharmacologists, pathologists, psychiatrists, general practitioners and epidemiologists (specialists in disease patterns in populations)? It may be covered in formal lectures and it will figure in discussion of individual patients in clinical teaching. Although many medical schools arrange some formal teaching about alcohol, very few attempt to integrate the disparate elements.

Behavioural scientists and psychologists are only occasionally involved, and the cultural and behavioural significance of alcohol is not considered. Helping individuals with alcohol-related problems should involve co-operation with many other disciplines such as specialist alcohol counsellors, social workers, probation officers and community alcohol team workers. However, these non-medical disciplines are rarely given the opportunity to contribute to the teaching of medical students about alcohol. The majority of teaching appears to adopt a predominantly medical model. It fails to explore other models of drinking behaviour or to examine concepts which blur the borders between normal and abnormal. This pattern of teaching is likely to lead to medical students adopting attitudes to alcohol which are curative and palliative rather than preventive and promotive.

Most of the cases seen in hospital will feature drinkers who have already suffered severe damage, while relatively little attention is paid to those who have only experienced slight and readily reversible problems. Teaching in general practice will allow the students to see a whole range of drinking behaviour, and to understand the opportunities for intervention at an early stage. General practice is also the ideal setting for observing shared care between the primary care team, other professionals and the family and for observing the management of conditions which tend to be chronic and may be lifelong. The problems posed by alcohol provide excellent material for multi-disciplinary teaching and can be used to illustrate many aspects of medical practice.[10, 11, 12] Teaching on alcohol should not be solely concerned with facts and skills, but should offer students the opportunity to explore their own attitudes and behaviour towards alcohol.[13] This helps students think about their own use of alcohol now and in the future, and also helps them appreciate the relationship between their own attitudes and behaviour and their responsibilities towards their patients.

Attitudes are learned rather than taught and the formal curriculum has a limited but important role. Seminars and discussion groups can contribute to value clarification and are a useful technique for exploring attitudes to alcohol use and to individuals with alcohol problems. Multidisciplinary workshops with specialist alcohol counsellors and other non-medical disciplines can be particularly helpful for exploring and challenging students' attitudes. The student is, however, much more likely to be influenced by the prevailing norms and culture around him. The medical school bar which sells alcohol at lunchtime, the host who laughs at a student who declines an alcoholic drink and the consultants who talk about patients with alcohol-related problems as non-deserving all say more about what the medical school regards as acceptable standards than do many hours of formal teaching.

Examination content is a powerful influence on the direction and effort of medical students. Examinations are seen as a statement of the importance attached by the medical school to each subject. If students are to place full value upon teaching about problems with alcohol then the final examinations and/or in-course assessments must include assessments related to that subject.[14]

Co-ordinated multidisciplinary teaching does not happen unless some named individual in the medical school takes responsibility for making it happen. Often that person will be in the psychiatry department, the department of general practice or the department of public health medicine but the essential requirement is that they should be committed to the work.

> *Recommendation No. 49*
>
> It is recommended that all medical schools should review the content of their curriculum to ensure that it gives due weight to prevention and management of alcohol-related problems. The teaching should not be exclusively hospital-based and non-medical disciplines should contribute to the teaching. The different elements of alcohol teaching throughout the course should be co-ordinated.

> *Recommendation No. 50*
>
> It is recommended that medical schools should examine the non-curricular aspects of medical school life to ensure that they are promoting healthy attitudes to alcohol use and that it is consistent with the attitudes being taught in the formal curriculum.

## ▶ Higher professional training

Good undergraduate training on alcohol-related problems will have to be reinforced in higher professional training which offers considerable scope for alcohol education.[15] The general practitioner is likely to encounter many patients with alcohol-related problems or high-risk drinking patterns, and their training must equip them to help these patients. Most vocational training schemes for general practice give time to the counselling and consulting skills which are needed. A number of training manuals and attitudinal questionnaires are also available.[16, 17, 18] Trainee general practitioners need to acquire experience of dealing with drinking problems in a supportive environment.

*Recommendation No. 51*

It is recommended that organisers of vocational training schemes for general practice should ensure that their courses cover the recognition and management in general practice of patients with alcohol-related problems or high-risk drinking patterns.

*Recommendation No. 52*

It is recommended that postgraduate tutors should ensure that higher medical training for physicians, surgeons, psychiatrists and public health physicians in their localities give adequate coverage to recognition and management of alcohol-related problems.

## ▶ Continuing education

The main objective of continuing education is to equip the doctor with new knowledge and new skills as they emerge during professional life. This 'retooling' is only part of a process of continuing education.[19] A second objective of continuing education is to improve the quality of clinical medicine by ensuring that knowledge and skills are also properly applied. Continuing education should help doctors retain the freshness and enthusiasm that characterises their first few years in post for the furthertwenty-five or thirty years of professional life.

Most doctors are keen to improve the quality of their clinical practice, including care of patients with alcohol-related problems. In order to do this they need practical assistance and not vague exhortations to translate good intentions into better practice. If it is to be effective, continuing education about alcohol must be acceptable to most doctors and not just to a few. A 5 per cent improvement in the effectiveness of the majority would have a far greater effect on public health than a 10 per cent improvement in the effectiveness of the keenest, or a 200 per cent in the effectiveness of the worst.

All doctors need continuing education but general practitioners, because they tend to be more isolated from their peers, may find it more difficult to arrange than hospital doctors. Continuing education on alcohol may involve all the usual study techniques, including seminars and lectures (which may be backed up with newsletters), group learning and study at home. Teaching which is coupled with the regular clinical work of the doctor is likely to be especially effective. Referral of the patient to a specialist alcohol worker, and the specialist's reply, offer a common and important opportunity for continuing education. There are ways in which doctors can be helped to learn at such teachable moments, for example by the provision of telephone 'hot lines', easy access to information (computer databases), and expert systems to help decision making.

Doctors not only need information about alcohol-related problems but also feedback about their own performance in managing those problems. Comparison of their performance with that of their peers and with accepted good practice is very powerful in modifying clinical behaviour. Such comparisons are even more likely to have an effect if the physicians themselves are involved in defining what constitutes good practice.

One hopeful innovation in continuing education is the introduction of 'facilitators'. These facilitators visit general practitioners and bring practical offers of assistance, which makes a welcome change from vague exhortations by distant authorities. The use of facilitators in encouraging assessment of risk factor status for coronary heart disease in general practice has been described and shown to be effective in a controlled trial.[20, 21] This model is now being applied to the screening for alcohol consumption and management of alcohol problems in primary care.

*Recommendation No. 53*

It is recommended that postgraduate tutors should ensure that both hospital doctors and general practitioners have opportunities through continuing education to refresh and update their skills in recognising and managing patients with alcohol-related problems.

## ▶ Changing public attitudes

Educational change and the provision of a supportive environment at best provide only a partial answer to doctors' difficulties in managing alcohol problems. At worst, by emphasising the centrality of the medical response to alcohol problems they divert attention from the importance of extraneous political and social factors on public health. It is unrealistic to expect doctors to respond enthusiastically to the task of detecting and managing alcohol problems while political and economic interests sustain public beliefs and attitudes towards drinking, which make it difficult for doctors and patients alike to acknowledge the existence of an alcohol problem.

## ▶ The exemplar role of the doctor

It is natural that doctors should feel uncomfortable with the idea of being required to set an example, but if they are to make a contribution to reducing alcohol-related harm it is unavoidable. The need for the doctor to be an example of safer drinking has recently been re-emphasised by the Royal College of Psychiatrists.[22] The previous paragraph pointed out the need for a change in public attitudes. Doctors cannot expect to be exempt and must be prepared to give a lead. It is not acceptable that the medical profession should be open to a charge of operating double standards.[23]

Adoption of an exemplar role is also necessary to help patients with alcohol-related problems. It is widely believed that the knowledge that most doctors had given up smoking was one of the factors that influenced so many smokers to stop. A doctor who is known to be a heavy drinker cannot expect to be a credible source for patients when counselling them to adopt safer drinking habits.

The Medical Royal Colleges and the British Medical Association must be vigilant to ensure that their corporate practice is consistent with their public pronouncements on alcohol. At every function where alcohol is offered they should ensure that equally attractive non-alcoholic alternatives are also available. It is a small gesture, but it demonstrates that they take their own rhetoric seriously.

## ▶ Other occupations

Doctors are not the only profession who are expected, as part of their work, to recognise and help people with alcohol-related problems. Nurses[24, 25] social workers and the other caring professions also have this role and therefore need to pay particular attention to drinking problems when they occur in their own professions. Nor are doctors the only group for whom it has been suggested that alcohol problems are an occupational hazard. The high rates of cirrhosis in certain other occupations (see Figure 11.1), suggest that alcohol-related problems may be common to them.

In this chapter the authors have chosen to concentrate on doctors because they themselves are doctors. Having experienced medical training and worked for many years with medical colleagues the authors felt justified in talking about the needs of their own profession and we leave it to those who have detailed knowledge of training and working situations in other professions to make recommendations about the needs of those professions.

FIGURE 11.1   *Liver cirrhosis deaths among British males for different occupations*

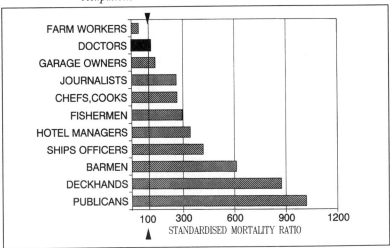

Average SMR is 100

SOURCE   M. A. Plant, *Drugs in Perspective* (London: Hodder & Stoughton, 1987), table 6.2.

References

1. P. Anderson, 'Managing alcohol problems in general practice', *British Medical Journal*, 290(1985) pp. 1873–5.
2. G. Lloyd, 'Alcoholic doctors can recover', *British Medical Journal*, 300(1990) pp. 728–30.
3. R. M. Murray, 'Alcoholism amongst male doctors in Scotland', *Lancet*, 2(1976) pp. 729–31.
4. M. Plant, *Drugs in perspective* (London: Hodder and Stoughton, 1989)
5. F. Adshead and A. W. Clare, 'Doctors' double standards on alcohol', *British Medical Journal*, 293(1986) pp. 1590–1.
6. J. Rucinski and F. Cybulska, 'Mentally ill doctors', *British Journal of Hospital Medicine*, 33(1985) pp. 90–4.
7. R. M. Murray, 'Characteristics and prognosis of alcoholic doctors', *British Medical Journal*, 2(1976) pp. 1537–9.
8. D. J. Collier and I. L. P. Beales, 'Drinking among medical students: a questionnaire survey', *British Medical Journal*, 299(1989) pp. 19–21.
9. Department of Health and Social Security, *Alcohol-related problems in undergraduate medical education. A survey of English medical schools* (London: DHSS, 1987).
10. A. D. Pokorny and J. Solomon, 'A follow-up survey of drug abuse and alcoholism teaching in medical schools', *Journal of Medical Education*, 58(1983) pp. 316–21.
11. M. J. Hanlon, 'A review of the recent literature relating to the training of medical students in alcoholism', *Journal of Medical Education*, 60(1985) pp. 618–26.
12. M. J. Ashby, S. Holt, H. Skinner, J. R. Peachey and J. G. Rankin, *Alcohol and drug-related problems* (University of Toronto, 1987).
13. A. W. Clare, 'Alcohol Education and the Medical Student', *Alcohol and Alcoholism*, 19(1984) pp. 291–6.
14. Association of University Teachers in General Practice, *Undergraduate Medical Education in General Practice*, Occasional Paper 28 (London: Royal College of General Practitioners, 1984).
15. DHSS, *Alcohol-related problems in higher professional and postgraduate medical education* (London: DHSS, 1987).
16. Royal College of General Practitioners, *Alcohol – A Balanced View* (London: Royal College of General Practitioners, 1986).
17. P. Anderson and S. Clement, 'The AAPPQ revisited. The management of general practitioners' attitudes to alcohol problems', *British Journal of Addiction*, 82(1987) pp. 753–60.
18. World Health Organisation, *Drug Dependence and Alcohol - related problems. A manual for community health workers with Guidelines for Trainees* (Geneva: World Health Organisation, 1986).

19. J. A. M. Gray, 'Continuing Medical Education: Retooling and Renaissance', *Lancet*, i(1986) pp. 1261–2.
20. E. Fullard, G. Fowler and M. Gray, 'Facilitating Prevention in Primary Care', *British Medical Journal*, 289(1984) pp. 1585–7.
21. E. Fullard, G. Fowler and M. Gray, 'Promoting prevention in primary care: controlled trial of low technology, low cost approach', *British Medical Journal*, 294(1987) pp. 1080–2.
22. Royal College of Psychiatrists, *The doctor as examplar of safer drinking* (Cyclostylist) (London: Royal College of Psychiatrists, 1989).
23. F. Adshead and A. W. Clare, 'Doctors' double standards on alcohol', op. cit.
24. G. E. La Godna and M. J. Hendrix, 'Impaired nurses: a cost analysis', *Journal of Nursing Administration*, 19(1989) pp. 13–18.
25. P. G. Booth, 'Managing alcohol and drug abuse in the nursing profession', *Journal of Advanced Nursing*, 12(1987) pp. 625–30.

# ▶ 12 ▶ ▶ ▶ ▶ ▶ ▶ ▶ ▶ ▶ ▶ ▶ ▶

# RECOMMENDATIONS FOR ACTION

## ▶ Who should do what?

This report and the recommendations contained in it are intended to stimulate action. Many different departments, agencies and postholders can contribute to reducing alcohol-related harm to public health. Co-operation between agencies is frequently the key to success, but one agency usually has to take responsibility for leading and co-ordinating action. In this last chapter we consider the responsibilities of the different agencies.

## ▶ The Government

Action at a local level has to be supported by appropriate action at a national level. Legislation provides the framework within which local agencies such as police and magistrates work. Taxation policy and advertising regulations affect the amount of alcohol purchased. Central guidance and central funding levels constrain the ability of statutory and voluntary sector agencies to provide service at the local level. Many government departments have responsibility for taking action to reduce alcohol-related harm.

## ▶ The Department of Health

The Department of Health has responsibility for ensuring that district health authorities provide a proper range of services for prevention and management of alcohol-related problems. They also have responsibility for ensuring that adequate funding is available for provision of these services. They need to have a clear strategy for reducing the harm to public health from alcohol (Recommendations 6 and 7, page 55); to collect better information (Recommendations 1 and 2, page 32); to ensure that funds are available both to prevent alcohol-related problems (Recommendation 13, page 76); and to provide services for those with such problems (Recommendation 34, page 149).

▶ The Treasury

Taxation is the responsibility of the Treasury and it could make a major contribution by considering public health when setting rates of duty on alcoholic drinks (Recommendations 17 and 18, page 104; Recommendations 19 and 20, page 105; and Recommendation 21, page 106). The Treasury should also obtain better information on the costs and benefits of alcohol to the economy (Recommendation 5, page 50).

▶ The Home Office

The Home Office has responsibility to ensure that public health is taken into consideration in licensing law, that the Courts and Prison Service deal constructively with offenders with alcohol-related problems and that the police and Probation Service prevent alcohol-related offences and disorder.

The Home Office should be taking the necessary actions to ensure that we have a better understanding of the link between alcohol and disorder (Recommendation 3, page 44), and that licensing law gives due weight to the public interest (Recommendation 16, page 91). It should also be taking steps to ensure that sentencing policy (Recommendation 42, page 166) and after-care of offenders (Recommendation 43, page 175) play their part in helping those whose offence was alcohol-related to find solutions to their drinking problems.

▶ The Department of Transport

The Department of Transport is responsible for promoting legislation in relation to drinking and driving. It should

197

redouble its efforts to get across the message that if one has to drive, don't drink alcohol (Recommendation 22, page 115; Recommendation 25, page 121; and Recommendation 31, page 132). Legislation and police powers should be amended to increase the likelihood that drink-drivers will be caught (Recommendations 23 and 24, page 120). Arrangements should be made both to stop drink-drive offenders from driving (Recommendation 26, page 124) and to help them resolve their alcohol-related problems before regaining their licence (Recommendation 28, page 130).

## ▶ The Ministry of Agriculture, Fisheries and Food

The Ministry of Agriculture, Fisheries and Food should regulate packaging of alcoholic drinks so that consumers are not misled as to the effects of these products and can easily assess how much alcohol they are consuming. (Recommendation 45, page 176 and Recommendation 46, page 177). It should also regulate advertising of alcohol so as to limit pressures to increase consumption (Recommendation 47, page 180 and Recommendation 48, page 181).

## ▶ The Health Education Authority

The Health Education Authority is charged with the duty of planning and carrying out health education in conjunction with district health authorities and local authorities. It has a responsibility to ensure that the public are properly informed about alcohol and should encourage health education programmes that use a variety of methods to stress the need to limit consumption and promote sensible drinking, through both individual and community decisions (Recommendation 6, page 55; Recommendations 8 and 9, page 66; Recommendation 10, page 71; Recommendation 22, page 115). Such activities need to be properly evaluated (Recommendation 11, page 71) and adequately funded (Recommendation 13, page 76).

## ▶ The BBC and IBA

The BBC and IBA have a duty to bear in mind the likely effect of their programmes on public health (Recommendation 12, page 75). The IBA also has a duty to ensure that alcohol advertising on television conforms to acceptable standards (Recommendation 47, page 180).

## ▶ The District Health Authorities and Family Health Service Authorities

Hospital services and community services managed by the district health authorities and general practice co-ordinated by the family health authorities (formerly known as family practitioner committees) ought to play major parts in preventing alcohol-related problems and in helping patients who have suffered alcohol-related harm. These authorities need more information on how alcohol affects demand for their services (Recommendation 2, page 32) and a clear strategy for preventing alcohol-related harm to public health (Recommendations 6 and 7, page 55 and Recommendation 34, page 149). The strategy needs to cover primary prevention (Recommendations 8 and 9, page 66; Recommendation 10, page 71; Recommendation 33, page 146; Recommendation 39, page 163 and Recommendation 40, page 164), and provision of service to those who have suffered alcohol-related harm (Recommendation 32, page 145; Recommendation 34, page 149; and Recommendation 41, page 166). In providing these services the health authorities and family practitioner committees will work closely with local authority departments, voluntary agencies, police, probation and other local agencies (Recommendations 35 and 36, page 157).

## ▶ Local authorities

The local authorities provide a wide range of services. Some departments (for example, social services and housing) come into contact with clients with alcohol-related problems. Other departments (for example, youth services and environmental services) offer opportunities for alcohol education. Yet other departments (catering, leisure services, and so on) manage licensed premises. Like the health authorities, the local authorities need better information on how alcohol affects demand for these services (Recommendation 4, page 47) and to have a consistent approach to the prevention of alcohol-related problems (Recommendations 6 and 7, page 55; Recommendation 35, page 157). They need to work in close co-operation with other local agencies (Recommendation 35 and 36, page 157; Recommendation 40, page 164; and Recommendation 41, page 166) and to ensure that all their activities are consistent with limiting alcohol-related harm (Recommendation 38, page 161; Recommendation 39, page 163).

## ▶ Local education authorities and schools

Local education authorities and schools have a responsibility to educate young people about alcohol (Recommendations 8 and 9, page 66; and Recommendation 37, page 159).

## ▶ Magistrates

Magistrates have a responsibility to ensure that offenders who have alcohol-related problems are encouraged to seek help with any underlying drink problem (Recommendation 28, page 130; Recommendation 42, page 166; and Recommendation 43, page 167).

## ▶ The Licensing Bench

Magistrates on the Licensing Bench are responsible for the local administration of licensing law and should bear in mind the health consequences of licensing decisions (Recommendation 14, page 90; Recommendation 16, page 91; and Recommendation 44, page 175) and make clear their concern over those who supply alcohol to drivers (Recommendation 27, page 125).

## ► The police

The police are responsible for enforcement of licensing law, prevention of drink-drive offences and prevention of other offences, disorder and nuisance related to alcohol use. They need better information on the association between alcohol and crime (Recommendation 3, page 44). Their powers to enforce drink-drive legislation need to be clarified (Recommendations 23 and 24, page 120; Recommendation 27, page 125 They also need clear policies on the enforcement of licensing law (Recommendation 15, page 90). They should work in close co-operation with other local agencies involved in preventing alcohol-related harm to public health and order (Recommendations 35 and 36, page 157).

## ► The Probation Service

In the course of their work the Probation Service have many opportunities to help offenders who have alcohol-related problems. They need a clear strategy for reducing alcohol-related harm (Recommendations 6 and 7, page 55) and working in conjunction with other local agencies (Recommendations 35 and 36, page 157). They have a particular role in helping offenders with alcohol-related problems (Recommendation 28, page 130; Recommendation 42, page 166; and Recommendation 43, page 167).

## ► Health education departments

Health education departments have responsibility to try and inform people in their locality about alcohol and drinking. They need a strategy aimed at both the general population and high risk groups (Recommendations 6 and 7, page 55) and they should use a variety of methods (Recommendations 8 and 9, page 66; Recommendations 10 and 11, page 71; Recommendation 13, page 76; Recommendation 22, page 115; Recommendation 40, page 164; and Recommendation 41, page 166). Health education departments should co-operate closely with other local agencies (Recommendations 35 and 36, page 157).

## ▶ Specialist alcohol agencies

Specialist alcohol agencies have a responsibility to ensure that their services are as accessible and acceptable as possible to all groups in the community (Recommendation 41, page 166) and form part of an integrated plan of service delivery. They need a shared strategy of prevention (Recommendations 6 and 7, page 55) and to work in close co-operation with the statutory agencies (Recommendations 35 and 36, page 157; and Recommendation 40, page 164).

## ▶ The alcohol trade

The alcohol trade has a responsibility to try and limit the harms associated with the consumption of the product they sell: there are ways of doing this without damaging their commercial interests (Recommendation 29, page 131; Recommendation 44, page 175; Recommendation 45, page 176; and Recommendation 46, page 177). It may also be necessary to further limit advertising and sponsorship by the alcohol industry (Recommendation 47, page 180; and Recommendation 48, page 181) in the interests of public health.

## ▶ Employers

Employers can reduce alcohol-related problems in their employees and the workplace by adopting a realistic workplace alcohol policy (Recommendation 30, page 132 and Recommendation 39, page 163).

## ▶ Medical schools and organisers of postgraduate medical education

All those involved in undergraduate or postgraduate medical education have a responsibility to ensure that doctors' training enables them to help prevent and to treat alcohol-related disease, which is both common and preventable. Medical teachers need to be clearer about strategies for reducing alcohol-related harm (Recommendations 6 and 7, page 55). They should review undergraduate and postgraduate education (Recommendations 49 and 50, page 189; Recommendations 51 and 52, page 190; and Recommendation 53, page 191) to remedy the weaknesses in medical education on alcohol-related harm.

## ▶ Everyone

We all have a responsibility to think about our own drinking behaviour and ensure that it does not place at risk either our own health or the health and well being of others.

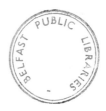

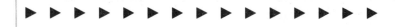

# USEFUL ADDRESSES

**Alcohol Concern**
Aims to stimulate and co-ordinate prevention work. Publishes *A Directory of Alcohol Services*. Produces a bi-monthly journal. Maintains a collection of books and other resources.
305 Gray's Inn Road, London WC1X 8QF
Telephone:  (071) 8333471.

**Institute of Alcohol Studies**
A source of information, and an organiser of education and training programmes for workers dealing with alcohol-related problems.
Alliance House, 12 Caxton Street, London SW1H 0GS
Telephone:  (071) 222 4001/5880.

**Social Insurance and Welfare Department, Trades Union Council**
Produces a set of recommendations on policies entitled *Problem Drinking: TUC Guidelines for a work place policy*.
Congress House, Great Russell Street, London WC1B 3LS
Telephone:  (071) 636 4030

**The Samaritans**
17 Uxbridge Road, Slough, Buerks
Telephone:  (0753) 32713

**Relate**
Herbert Gray College, Little Church Street, Rugby CV21 3AP
Telephone:  (0788) 73241)

**Alcoholics Anonymous**
11 Redcliffe Gardens, London SW10 9BQ
Telephone:  (071) 352 9779

**Al Anon/Al Ateen**
Al-Anon, 61 Great Dover Street, London SE1 4YF
Telephone: (071) 403 0888

**Health and Safety at Work. Central Office.**
Institute of Occupation Safety and Health (IOSH)
222 Uppingham Road, Leicester LE5 0QG

**Health Education Authority**
Hamilton House, Mabledon Place, London WC1H 9TX
Telephone: (071) 383 3833

**Standing Conference on Drug Abuse**
1–4 Hatton Place, Hatton Garden, London EC1N 8ND
Telephone: (071) 430 2341

**Medical Council on Alcoholism**
1 St Andrew's Place, London NW1 4LB
Telephone: (071) 487 4445

**TACADE (Teacher's Advisory Council on Alcohol and Drug Education)**
2 Mount Street, Manchester M2 5NG
Telephone: (061) 834 7210

**DAWN (Drugs, Alcohol, Women Nationally)**
Boundary House, 91–92 Charterhouse Street, London
EC1M 6HL
Telephone: (071) 250 3280

**Turning Point**
National charity with projects throughout the country.
CAP House, 9/12 Long Lane, London EC1A 9HA
Telephone: (071) 606 3947

**Aquarius**
Charity with projects throughout the Midlands.
The White House, 111 New Street, Birmingham B24EU
Telephone: (021) 632 4727

**Salvation Army**
Runs a number of projects (particularly hostels) for homeless people.
101 Queen Victoria Street, London EC4P 3EP
Telephone: (071) 236 5224

Scotland

## Scottish Council on Alcoholism
147 Blythswood Street, Glasgow G2 4EN
Telephone: (041) 333 9677

## Scottish Health Education Group
Woodburn House, Canaan Lane, Edinburgh EH10 4SG
Telephone: (031) 447 8044

Northern Ireland

## Northern Ireland Council on Alcohol
40 Elmwood Avenue, Belfast BT9 6AZ
Telephone: (0232) 664434

## Council on Alcohol Related Problems
12 Lombard Street, Belfast BT1 1RD
Telephone: (0232) 224176

## Northern Ireland Health Education Authority
Dundonald House, Upper Newtonards Road, Belfast
Telephone: (0232) 650111

Wales

## Health Promotion Authority for Wales
8th Floor, Brunel House, 2 Fitzalan Road, Cardiff CF2 1EB
Telephone: (0222) 472472

## Alcohol Concern (Wales)
9th Floor, Brunel House, 2 Fitzalan Road, Cardiff CF2 1EB
Telephone: (0222) 488002

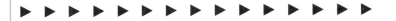

# INDEX